Ungoverned and Out of Sight

UNGOVERNED AND OUT OF SIGHT

Public Health and the Political Crisis of Homelessness in the United States

Charley E. Willison

OXFORD
UNIVERSITY PRESS

Oxford University Press is a department of the University of Oxford. It furthers the University's objective of excellence in research, scholarship, and education by publishing worldwide. Oxford is a registered trade mark of Oxford University Press in the UK and certain other countries.

Published in the United States of America by Oxford University Press
198 Madison Avenue, New York, NY 10016, United States of America.

Library of Congress Cataloging-in-Publication Data
Names: Willison, Charley E., author.
Title: Ungoverned and out of sight : public health and the political crisis
of homelessness in the United States / Charley E. Willison.
Description: New York, NY : Oxford University Press, [2021] |
Includes bibliographical references and index.
Identifiers: LCCN 2020048680 (print) | LCCN 2020048681 (ebook) |
ISBN 9780197548325 (paperback) | ISBN 9780197548349 (epub) |
ISBN 9780197548356 (online)
Subjects: MESH: Homeless Persons | Public Health | Health Policy |
Politics | United States
Classification: LCC RA418.5.P6 (print) | LCC RA418.5.P6 (ebook) |
NLM WA 300 AA1 | DDC 362.1086/942—dc23
LC record available at https://lccn.loc.gov/2020048680
LC ebook record available at https://lccn.loc.gov/2020048681

DOI: 10.1093/oso/9780197548325.001.0001

This material is not intended to be, and should not be considered, a substitute for medical or other professional advice. Treatment for the conditions described in this material is highly dependent on the individual circumstances. And, while this material is designed to offer accurate information with respect to the subject matter covered and to be current as of the time it was written, research and knowledge about medical and health issues is constantly evolving and dose schedules for medications are being revised continually, with new side effects recognized and accounted for regularly. Readers must therefore always check the product information and clinical procedures with the most up-to-date published product information and data sheets provided by the manufacturers and the most recent codes of conduct and safety regulation. The publisher and the authors make no representations or warranties to readers, express or implied, as to the accuracy or completeness of this material. Without limiting the foregoing, the publisher and the authors make no representations or warranties as to the accuracy or efficacy of the drug dosages mentioned in the material. The authors and the publisher do not accept, and expressly disclaim, any responsibility for any liability, loss, or risk that may be claimed or incurred as a consequence of the use and/or application of any of the contents of this material.

9 8 7 6 5 4 3 2 1

Printed by Marquis, Canada

CONTENTS

ACKNOWLEDGMENTS

When I chose homeless policy as a research topic for my dissertation, I never anticipated the challenges that would come along with it. This was a demanding book to write, in many ways, because this topic lies at the intersection of many different issues in health and public health policy and is simultaneously omitted from most health policy research and debates. I encountered the question, "Why is homelessness a health problem?" from health policy scholars often throughout this process. I also often received dismay when discussing problems related to policing and homelessness.

The lessons I learned writing this book certainly apply to existing challenges in homeless policy and homeless policy governance. Homelessness is an uncomfortable subject that has often been overlooked, formally and informally, in public health and social policy spaces. I am writing these acknowledgments during the Covid-19 pandemic and the global unrest in response to the police killings of unarmed Black Americans. The pandemic is and will continue to affect rates of homelessness in extreme ways. The waves of protest are bringing to the fold the reality of policing in America. If there was ever a time to acknowledge the challenges related to homelessness and homeless policy in the United States, 2020 is about time.

There are many people I would like to thank who helped make this book possible. First and foremost, thank you to my dissertation committee at the University of Michigan. Scott Greer and Holly Jarman were incredible advisors and committee chairs who took a chance on me as a nontraditional student and a chance on this research topic. Scott and Holly never faltered in their support for the work I was doing and continually made it stronger. I am incredibly grateful to Chuck Shipan, Nick Bagley, and Rebecca Haffajee for their mentorship and thoughtful contributions that notably improved the research.

The University of Michigan was a wonderful place to study health politics. There are too many professors in the School of Public Health and the Department of Political Science for me to name everyone, but I would like to give special thanks to a couple faculty who became valued mentors and collaborators: Julia Wolfson and Melissa Creary. Thank you, too, to the Department of Political Science Interdisciplinary Workshop in American Politics and the American Institutions Group, led by Chuck Shipan, that provided valuable feedback and engagement.

I made so many wonderful friends at Michigan who provided invaluable emotional and social support in addition to rigorous feedback on my research. I am particularly grateful for collaborations with Phil Singer, Denise Lillvis, and Amanda Mauri, who helped work through various components of this research and provided incredible feedback. Big thanks to Phil Singer, who read different drafts of the manuscript chapters.

I am grateful to many additional scholars outside the University of Michigan who provided important support and insight along the way. In particular, I thank David Jones, who walked me through the steps of writing a dissertation and then a book, from beginning to end. I am also very grateful to Katherine Levine Einstein, who has provided mentorship and guidance to ground this research in urban politics. I am also incredibly grateful for being a part of the American Political Science Association Health Politics Working Group, which has been an immense source of insight, encouragement, and inspiration.

Thank you to the many mentors, colleagues, and friends at Harvard University who have been extremely supportive. In particular, Haiden Huskamp, who brought me to the Harvard Department of Health Care Policy for this fellowship and offered regular encouragement, and advice throughout the publication process. Thank you to Richard Frank and the Harvard Initiative on Health and Homelessness for providing community in my scholarship and reinforcement of its importance. Thank you to Benjamin Cook and all of my friends and colleagues at the Harvard Health Equity Research Lab for being a sounding board for my research and supporting me through the process. Thank you to the Harvard Department of Government for bringing me into the American Politics community and to the Scholars Strategy Network for offering new avenues to disseminate this research.

I am grateful for funding received from a variety of sources that made this research possible, including grants and fellowships from the Rackham Graduate School at the University of Michigan, the Agency for Healthcare Research and Quality doctoral traineeship, Harold and Vivian Shapiro Award, Martha and Ernest Hammel Award, and grants from the Center for the Education of Women and the Department of Health Management and Policy at the University of Michigan, and the National Institutes of Mental Health Postdoctoral Fellowship.[1]

Thank you to everyone I interviewed for this project and the many people who pointed me in the right direction to locate primary policy documents. This book would not have been possible without these contributions. Special thanks to the San Francisco History Center, the Online Archive of California, the Ronald Reagan Presidential Library, and Shreveport City Hall. I also thank Sarah Humprehville at Oxford University Press and the two anonymous reviewers whose feedback helped me improve the manuscript.

Most important, I thank my family. My mother, Melanie Willison, along with my second family, Jill, Randy, Jacqui, Zack, and Randall Hoyle, are a constant source of support, inspiration, and love. I am grateful for the unending love and support from my cats Atlas and Cosmos, and my dog, Cleo. And of course, thank you to my husband, Gurhari Singh, who provided unending encouragement and valuable critique throughout this research and continues to support all my endeavors. I dedicate this work to my father, David Willison, who was a great source of inspiration and support.

CHAPTER 1

America's Homelessness Crisis

HOMELESSNESS IS A PUBLIC HEALTH PROBLEM

Homelessness is a public health problem. From rising housing costs to discriminatory lending and leasing, natural disasters, and mental illness, homelessness has many different causes and many similar effects: serious adverse consequences for physical and mental health, quality of life, and educational and work attainment. In the public health and medical communities, there is a resounding call to promote a culture of health across communities and "health in all" policies. Yet, the national conversation around health reform centers on healthcare, including health insurance and medical care. Often conspicuously absent from these debates are factors influencing population health across the life course.

Homelessness, at its core, is a threat to population health and health equity. Nearly a decade after the Great Recession of 2008, homelessness rates are once again increasing across the United States (Bishop et al. 2017). Homelessness affects over 3.5 million young Americans annually (Chapin Hall University of Chicago 2018), of which 1.3 million are children (United States Interagency Council on Homelessness 2018).[1] This is more than the number of Americans who suffer annually from opioid-related substance use disorders (National Institute on Drug Abuse 2018) and more than the number of Americans who die in car accidents annually (Insurance Institute for Highway Safety and Highway Loss Data Institute 2018). Black Americans are four times as likely and Hispanic Americans are two times more likely to experience homelessness compared to white Americans (Fusaro, Levy, and Shaefer 2018). Among children, homelessness contributes to higher rates of developmental, academic, and behavioral problems (Grant et al. 2013).

Ungoverned and Out of Sight. Charley E. Willison, Oxford University Press (2021). © Oxford University Press.
DOI: 10.1093/oso/9780197548325.003.0001

Downstream across the life course, homelessness contributes to high rates of chronic disease, adverse behavioral health outcomes, increased mortality, and lower rates of educational and job attainment (Maxmen 2019). Longer durations of homelessness[2] are associated with higher mortality, rates of severe mental illness and substance use disorders, and chronic medical conditions; persons experiencing chronic homelessness are more likely to remain homeless as length of homelessness increases (Henwood, Byrne, and Scriber 2015; Kertesz et al. 2016) Ultimately, homelessness worsens health disparities for already vulnerable low-income and minority populations. If health policy truly seeks to improve population health and reduce health disparities, addressing homelessness must be a priority.

Cities are the face of the U.S. homeless epidemic. If you have traveled to San Francisco; Los Angeles; Washington, DC; or almost any major metropolitan area in the United States in recent years, you almost certainly encountered homelessness. With increasing visibility, homelessness paints a stark image of inequality in modern America. In Los Angeles, over 35,000 individuals are experiencing homelessness (Cowan 2019). Rates of unsheltered homelessness, or primarily long-term homelessness,[3] increased by over 40% in recent years in Los Angeles alone (Cowan 2019). Nationally, unsheltered homelessness grew at a rate of 3%, and chronic or long-term homelessness by 9% over the past two years (U.S. Department of Housing and Urban Development 2019a). Simultaneously, mortality rates of individuals experiencing long-term homelessness in cities across the United States are increasing dramatically (Gorman and Rowan 2019; Maxmen 2019). What are municipalities doing to respond to this crisis? This book seeks to measure and explain *local responses* to homelessness, or local homeless policy decision-making, as the main outcome of interest, focusing on municipal management of long-term or chronic homelessness.

HOMELESS POLICY GOVERNANCE IN THE UNITED STATES

There are many different approaches to managing public health crises. The most common approach leverages governmental intervention. Anyone who works in public health will tell you that local-level public health departments are a critical part of public health infrastructure for both prevention and disaster response. Local public health departments are responsible for many different population health activities including adult and child immunizations, screening and treatment for chronic and communicable diseases or conditions including behavioral health, and maternal and child health services. Municipal housing departments, often working with local public health departments, work to coordinate resources and services to provide affordable, safe, quality housing to residents. In the context of disasters themselves, natural or health, disaster governance protocol stemming from federated powers outlined in Article 10 of the constitution emphasizes the role of local governments as first responders in such crises followed by support from states and the federal government (Federal Emergency Management Agency 2003).

Yet in homeless policy, the systems governing homelessness and designing and delivering homeless policy in the United States typically do not include local governments (Jarpe, Mosely, and Smith 2019). The majority of homeless governance systems in the United States are overseen and directed by nonprofit organizations. Previous research has shown that only 38% of homeless governance systems in the United States are a part of municipal government (Jarpe, Mosely, and Smith 2019). The primarily nonprofit, nongovernmental systems governing homelessness in the United States are known as Continuums of Care. The U.S. Department of Housing and Urban Development (HUD; 2017b) definition of the Continuum of Care is as follows:

> *Continuum of Care and Continuum* means the group organized to carry out the responsibilities required under this part and that is composed of representatives of organizations, including nonprofit homeless providers, victim service providers, faith-based organizations, governments, businesses, advocates, public housing agencies, school districts, social service providers, mental health agencies, hospitals, universities, affordable housing developers, law enforcement, organizations that serve homeless and formerly homeless veterans, and homeless and formerly homeless persons to the extent these groups are represented within the geographic area and are available to participate.

More generally, the Continuums of Care, or the national system for preventing and addressing homelessness in the United States, are a network of mainly nongovernmental community organizations, arranged at the municipal level that distribute funding and oversee local and regional homeless policy programming and service distribution. This primarily decentralized model—or shifting governance entirely to nongovernmental actors—of governance for homeless policy is unique among health and social services policy governance structures.

Most research on homelessness focuses on empirical research identifying best practices for solutions to chronic or long-term homelessness. However, there is a wide gap in the literature investigating the political processes shaping the reality of establishing or implementing these best practices. This book seeks to understand the political processes influencing adoption of best-practice solutions to reduce chronic homelessness, or homeless policy decision-making, in municipalities across the United States.

As discussed, homelessness is a unique case of a health issue that is governed by an almost entirely decentralized system—both historically and today (Jarpe, Mosely, and Smith 2019). The history of devolution and decentralization in homelessness governance makes it a unique policy space where various actors compete and implement very different types of policies that all attempt to manage homelessness and long-term homelessness to different ends. This book applies a mixed methods, explanatory sequential design utilizing national data on local homeless policy choices and in-depth case studies in three cities—San Francisco, CA; Atlanta, GA; and Shreveport, LA—to explain divergent approaches to addressing long-term homelessness.

This book argues that homelessness policy, specifically policies seeking solutions to long-term or chronic homelessness, are governed by four separate and distinct policy interests: the state, local government, economic elites, and homeless service providers. The separation and conflict between these policy interests result in increased challenges to establishing and implementing effective policy solutions to end chronic homelessness. Challenges include limited state-level support such as financial resources and/or administrative burdens due to misaligned policy goals; inequity in political participation that may exclude at-risk populations or bias participation in favor of economic elites; and, finally, limited involvement by municipal governments in many cases, which may constrain homeless programming due to inherent funding limitations and service coordination barriers. Overall, the limited coordination between these policy arenas and the strong trend in decentralization in homeless policy governance contribute to fewer public policy alternatives and increase the policy alternatives for private actors.

To measure municipal approaches to chronic homelessness, or local homeless policy governance, this research focuses on the political decision-making regarding the adoption of, or not, supportive housing policies by municipalities across the United States as the dependent variable. Nearly four decades of research has demonstrated that permanent supportive housing—specifically Housing First, which provides housing without be-havioral prerequisites to housing access—is the most effective way to suc-cessfully end chronic homelessness permanently (M. M. Brown et al. 2016; Evans, Collins, and Anderson 2016; Greenwood, Stefancic, and Tsemberis 2013; Kirst et al. 2014; National Academies of Sciences Engineering and Medicine 2018; Stanhope and Dunn 2011).[4] Permanent supportive housing provides simultaneous access to both housing and supportive medical and behavioral health services for persons experiencing chronic homelessness. Providing housing allows individuals to feel safe and to access basic needs like sleep, food, and water, promoting an environment where individuals can, subsequently, successfully address chronic medical and behavioral health conditions (Kertesz et al. 2016; National Academies of Sciences Engineering and Medicine 2018). Housing First has been the only approach to chronic homelessness that has led to successful, long-term housing sta-bility (M. M. Brown et al. 2016; Leff et al. 2009; Palepu et al. 2013).

CONTINUUMS OF CARE AND INCREASING MUNICIPAL RELATIONS

Since 2015, the Continuums of Care have been required by federal funding to move toward adopting supportive housing with a Housing First ap-proach as their primary means to addressing homelessness (Goodloe 2015). At the same time, the Continuums of Care are also now required to take steps to reduce criminalization of, or reactionary law enforcement responses to, individuals experiencing chronic homelessness (T. Bauman et al. 2017; Tars 2015).[5] Criminalization of homelessness through policing responses directly conflict with supportive housing policy goals and imple-mentation, by addressing behaviors associated with homelessness instead of the causes of homelessness and, ultimately, redirecting individuals into the criminal justice system as opposed to health and social services leading to ongoing cycles of incarceration and homelessness, especially among per-sons experiencing chronic homelessness (Berkeley Law Policy Advocacy Clinic 2018; Hawthorne et al. 2012; Mcnamara, Crawford, and Burns 2013; McNiel, Binder, and Robinson 2005; Robinson 2019; Segal, Frasso, and Sisti 2018).

Both of these regulatory changes involve primary components of mu-nicipal governance, including policing and incarceration, and zoning and building permitting (for permanent supportive housing units as well as transitional shelter facilities in the interim of permanent supportive housing). To facilitate planning and success of these and other Continuum of Care policies, HUD has begun encouraging coordination between Continuums of Care and municipal governments, although this process is still voluntary (HUD Office of Policy Development and Research 2018). Thus, measuring political decision-making regarding municipal supportive housing policy provides an indication of the relative coordination between municipal governments, and Continuums of Care in their designated tasks to utilize best practices.

MUNICIPAL HOMELESS POLICY DECISION-MAKING

There are many reasons why municipal governments may or may not choose to engage in homeless policy governance, and specifically in evidence-based practice. Homeless policy decision-making is a policy space that has been shaped substantially by the ways persons experiencing homelessness and chronic homelessness have been socially constructed by political decision makers (Jones 2015). The ways that persons experiencing chronic homelessness are perceived may interact with the dynamics of political privilege arising from variation in economic power across stakeholder groups. The variation in economic power across stakeholders may also include policy capacity encompassing resources available to effectively design and implement supportive housing policy. This interaction may further inform the types of policies pursued by different groups. This may include more or less participation by local governments in response to local *perceptions* about the causes of chronic homelessness and local government's ability to act based on available policy capacity and facility to integrate that policy capacity into local decision-making structures.

Thus, as discussed, the key independent variables of interest in this research are *political factors*, related to the adoption of evidence-based practices at the municipal level to address chronic homelessness. These political factors include two primary categories: the role of political institutions—here, in particular, the influence of decentralization in political institutional arrangements that subsequently shape how actors are able to participate in local policy decisions—and the role of social construction of persons experiencing homelessness, or how perceptions of the policy target population may influence what policies are pursued by different groups and to what end. Homeless policy politics has important theoretical implications for our contemporary understandings of decentralization in public health governance, and the implications of decentralization for the politics of historically and contemporarily marginalized populations, and, ultimately, successful policy design and implementation.

THE HISTORY OF U.S. HOMELESS POLICY

To understand the current state of homeless policy in the United States and why the majority of Continuums of Care are not a part of local government, we must examine the history of U.S. homeless policy. Homelessness policy in the United States is an amalgamation of governmental decentralization and community choices. Homelessness has always been a problem, but a problem that was never really addressed by government until the mid-late 20th century (Grob 1994). It was, instead, a history of familial responsibility and community-based organizations seeking to manage an undesirable issue (Grob 1994; Jones 2015; National Coalition for the Homeless 2006). The current policy space reflects this history.

There is one federal policy that specifically addresses homelessness. This is the McKinney–Vento Homeless Assistance Act, now known as the Homeless Emergency Assistance and Rapid Transition to Housing (HEARTH) Act, as amended in 2009 (U.S. Department of Housing and Urban Development 2009). McKinney–Vento was passed in 1987 under the Reagan administration. The legislation was purposefully structured to prioritize municipal or community authority in allocating federal funding, as a way to diminish federal involvement in homelessness and reduce governmental authority (Cronley 2010; Dreier 2007).

The McKinney–Vento Act established the main network of service provision and funding distribution for homeless policies (U.S. Department of Housing and Urban Development 2012). This network is known as the Continuum of Care. As discussed, the Continuums of Care are a national network of historically nongovernmental community organizations that distribute funding and oversee local and regional homeless policy programming and service distribution. Not all homeless service providers belong to the Continuums of Care, but the Continuums of Care receive and manage federal homeless funding to distribute to local actors. Today, the Continuums of Care, in conjunction with municipal governments, develop and implement homeless policies.

METHODOLOGICAL APPROACH

Explaining municipal policy outcomes is a relatively overlooked area in health politics and public health policy analysis. Most often, researchers focus on state-level policy analysis, or the effects of federal decision-making on state-level choices. As a result, there are very limited data on municipal policy outcomes, particularly in research focusing on municipal health, social services, or welfare policy. Homelessness falls into this category. This book utilizes a mixed methods explanatory sequential design utilizing novel data—a unique data set I designed including 232 municipalities receiving federal funding to address homelessness representing two-thirds of Continuums of Care, paired with in-depth interviews and archival analysis of policy documents in three exemplar municipal case studies identified from the national data—to define the scope of the problem and subsequently interrogate explanations of divergent policy approaches to address chronic homelessness.

I am focusing on examining the influence of intergovernmental relations—in particular, decentralization—and social construction on these policy outcomes. Mixed methods research adapts to data-constrained scenarios, providing researchers multiple avenues to examine a research question, gather data, and apply inference strategies. In the case of a mixed methods, explanatory sequential design, this strategy begins with a quantitative approach and ends with a qualitative approach that is informed by the findings from the quantitative analysis. The key aspect of this design is that it is meant to be used in scenarios with data constraints or little previously existing research. To adapt to these limitations, the approach uses an initial *exploratory* quantitative component to gain critical information about the scope of the issue and relevant trends in the data. These descriptive data and predictive trends may shed light on the explanatory mechanisms later on when a causal inference strategy can be applied or may at least inform next steps and future research (Mahoney and Thelen 2015). This approach may be especially relevant in policy analysis, where the dependent variable or outcomes of interest present more measurement challenges, and natural experiments may not readily exist to control for policy adoption.

The next phase in the explanatory sequential approach addresses these issues. The quantitative stage is followed by *explanatory* qualitative analysis. Qualitative analysis allows researchers to gain more depth in their analyses to understand the explanatory mechanisms at work more completely, compared to variable-based approaches alone, which may oversimplify some mechanisms. Qualitative analysis is also particularly effective in policy and politics research, where causal mechanisms are very complex and interwoven and quantitative analysis may face data limitations or be too reductionist to outline a complete picture of the causal processes at work.

SUMMARY OF THE FINDINGS

Homelessness is a surprising case of a public health issue that is governed by a primarily decentralized system of nongovernmental actors—both historically and today. The history of devolution and decentralization in homelessness governance makes it a unique policy arena where various actors compete and implement very different types of policies, all attempting to manage homelessness and long-term homelessness to different ends. HUD has recently been encouraging partnerships between nongovernmental actors and local governments in homeless policy governance to help improve policy coordination and implementation. This book specifically investigates municipal responses to chronic homelessness emphasizing why municipal governments may or may not choose to formally engage in responses to chronic homelessness and why municipalities may or may not develop evidence-based policies.

This book argues that homelessness policy is a very fragmented and disjointed policy space as a result of decades of decentralization. Responses to chronic homelessness are governed in four separate and distinct policy arenas: the state, local government, elites, and homeless service providers, or the Continuum of Care. The separation and conflict between these governing approaches result in increased challenges to establishing and implementing effective policy solutions to end chronic homelessness. Challenges include (1) relatively limited state-level support such as financial resources and/or administrative burdens stemming from misaligned policy goals between state policies and Continuum of Care programming or the needs of persons experiencing homelessness on the ground; (2) inequity in political participation that may exclude at-risk populations or bias participation in favor of economic elites; and (3) limited involvement by municipal governments in many cases. When municipal governments remain absent from homeless governance, Continuums of Care may be constrained in their ability to carry out policies and programming as a result of insufficient funding or lack of coordination with local government required to provide other necessary services such as behavioral healthcare, Medicaid administration, policing and incarceration, and zoning for or constructing supportive housing units themselves. Ultimately, conflicting policy goals across the four policy arenas and decentralization of homelessness policy governance contribute to fewer publicly funded policy alternatives for solutions to chronic homelessness and increase the policy alternatives for private actors.

This research finds that growth in policy capacity paired with structural changes incentivizing recentralization of homelessness governance may be required to promote interaction and coordination across the policy approaches to overcome collective action problems and to develop and implement effective solutions to long-term homelessness. However, a persistent problem that may require solutions beyond integration of the Continuum of Care and municipal government is protection of minority group and policy target populations in homeless policy debates. Across all cases in the research, homeless policy decision-making typically excludes persons who are at-risk of homelessness or are currently or formerly homeless. This lack of responsiveness or bias in policy decision-making may promote implementation challenges by skewing processes in favor of elite preferences who generally oppose permanent supportive housing and may lead to policy adoption that does not successfully address the causes of chronic homelessness.

OUTLINE OF THE BOOK

In each chapter, the similarities and differences between municipalities with local supportive housing policies and those without are examined, and evidence is provided that even in municipalities with different policy outcomes—that is, those with and without local supportive housing policies—similar political logic and processes apply to decision-making in both policy adoption and implementation, leading to similar, persistent challenges in approaches to chronic homelessness across municipalities related to policy coordination and decentralization.

Chapter 2 reviews the empirical and theoretical literature informing our understanding of homeless policy development, including decentralization, neoliberalism, the local political economy, social construction, and criminalization. Public health as a discipline studies issues influenced by local politics and policies that are primarily implemented—and, in many cases, governed—by local-level public health departments. Yet the world of public health policy tends to focus on the politics and policies at the state and federal level. Obscuring the role of local politics and in designing and implementing public health policies inaccurately portrays the functioning of public health systems and can lead to incorrect or incomplete assumptions about the effects of health politics on public health outcomes. Homelessness is no exception. Homelessness is a policy space with a long history of expanded governing authority for communities and local governments. To understand policy outcomes in homelessness governance, we must draw from the theories of urban politics and inter-governmental relations that have been developed to explain social policy. Chapter 2 develops the main theoretical argument of the book: (1) the limited coordination between policy interests governing homeless policy and (2) strong trends of decentralization in homeless policy governance contribute to fewer publicly funded policy alternatives for solutions to chronic homelessness and increase the policy alternatives for private actors.

Chapter 3 describes the rationale for conducting a mixed methods, explanatory sequential design—that is, the use of quantitative data to first explore trends in an understudied subject, followed by in-depth qualitative analyses to explain the mechanisms behind the broader trends. Chapter 3 outlines the quantitative data, sample selection, and methodological approaches. A novel national data set was built to identify political characteristics associated with the presence of a municipal level supportive housing policy (Willison 2020). The sample includes municipalities receiving federal funding to address homelessness. Logistic regression is paired with set theoretic analyses to understand both mean trends and heterogeneity in the sample that average effects may otherwise obscure to understand the variations in characteristics across municipalities in each outcome set (Ragin 2015).

This chapter subsequently discusses the case selection strategy stemming from the results from the national analysis, and the qualitative methods and data. Three municipal cases were selected from the national data set to provide in-depth explanations of the mechanisms behind local choices to adopt, or not to adopt, supportive housing policy. The cases were chosen using a stratified, proportional sampling method in the set-theoretic analyses to capture cases representative of major trends in the national data. The three cases are San Francisco, CA; Atlanta, GA; and Shreveport, LA. Qualitative case studies are a useful approach to enhance understanding of policy decision-making processes because they provide inherent flexibility to use all relevant data and present it in a variety of ways (Anckar 2008). Applying rigorously selected cases and in-depth qualitative analyses enhance quantitative findings by further examining the complex relationships and temporality of multiple factors affecting policy decision-making (Anckar 2008). In each case, I collected two types of qualitative data: interviews and textual document data. Interviews and document analysis add contextual grounding of the complicated relationships between the multiple factors at work and help tease a part political decision-making processes, leading to the outcome with a greater level of detail (Collier 2011).

Chapter 4 examines the national variation in municipal responses to chronic homelessness. Specifically, the goals of this chapter are to (1) identify the prevalence of municipal-level supportive housing policies among municipalities affected by homelessness in the United States and (2) identify and examine the factors associated with the presence of a municipal-level supportive housing policy. From a public health perspective, the presence of municipal-level supportive housing policies is an indication of evidence-based policy adoption to effectively address chronic homelessness in urban areas. To date, there has been almost no research on the political predictors (or other social or economic predictors) of the adoption of these evidence-based policies. Research has shown that the number of supportive housing units is not correlated with homelessness prevalence (T. Byrne et al. 2014). This would suggest that other factors, such as political predictors of policy adoption and implementation, might be affecting supportive housing policy. This research intends to fill that gap. Results demonstrate that most municipalities facing homelessness challenges do not have supportive housing policies. Of the municipalities in the data set, only 40% had a municipal-level supportive housing policy. These municipalities tend to be more liberal, sanctuary cities, have fewer but better funded nonprofit health organizations and lower rates of municipal governmental fragmentation, and are located in states without Medicaid expansion—in short, in (relatively) liberal municipalities in Republican states.

Chapter 5 presents the case study results from San Francisco. San Francisco represents municipalities with a local supportive housing policy (see Chapter 3). San Francisco is an example of the significance of policy implementation as a critical process that cannot be overlooked when examining the success of policy initiatives. At first glance, San Francisco should be very well positioned to successfully tackle chronic homelessness compared to other cities across the United States. San Francisco has a strong municipal tax base that allows for local investments in social services that other municipalities are not able to provide. The liberal ideology of San Francisco has historically placed San Francisco on the forefront of innovatively tackling social problems related to chronic homelessness including HIV/AIDS and the provision of county-level behavioral health services. Finally, San Francisco has a municipally governed Continuum of Care (homeless governing system) that is supported by other strong, local social service and health programs including the Department of Public Health and the Human Services Agency. This position in local government allowed San Francisco's Continuum of Care to have improved ability to participate in municipal decision-making related to homelessness and provide the Continuum of Care with authority to successfully design and carryout local policies related to homelessness. This is an advantage compared to other decentralized counterparts across the United States that have little to no governing authority and are limited in their ability to coordinate with police, county public health agencies, and elected officials and to have a voice regarding municipal funding, zoning, or budget priorities.

Yet, despite all these characteristics that would seemingly place San Francisco at the pinnacle of success for supportive housing policy implementation, many of the Continuums of Care's efforts have been stagnated at the implementation phase as a result of elite interference and state-level administrative and funding constraints. San Francisco is a city with a very visible homelessness epidemic. The problem will not be solved until implementation problems can be overcome by improving participatory equity in political decision-making to include minorities and at-risk groups, limiting elected officials' ability to interfere with bureaucrats' duties to carryout supportive housing regulation, and improving state-level coordination with municipal goals to reduce administrative burdens and align funding mechanisms.

Chapter 6 presents the case study results from Atlanta. Atlanta, like San Francisco, represents municipalities with a supportive housing policy but diverges from San Francisco on a few key characteristics of interest (Atlanta's population is majority Black, and Georgia as a state has not expanded Medicaid). Atlanta is a case where the Continuum of Care has become integrated into municipal government and homeless policy processes. Atlanta also came to have a municipal supportive housing policy by way of institutional restructuring. Atlanta's reform occurred when the Continuum of Care restructured, moving from a tri-jurisdictional arrangement to separate city and county Continuums of Care. The restructuring was prefaced by an investment in homelessness and chronic homelessness prevention and services by the city of Atlanta. Since then, the city adopted a supportive housing policy and made the choice to oversee the new city of Atlanta Continuum of Care, integrating these policy processes.

Despite these policy changes Atlanta still suffers from serious barriers to policy implementation resulting from the histories of racism and segregation, entrenched elite preferences, and limited state involvement. There exists a strong, separate policy effort mobilizing police services to coordinate an indirect and informal policy space of moving groups of persons experiencing homelessness to other jurisdictions or away from desirable areas based on the desires of organized economic elites. Finally, Atlanta faces significant funding challenges related to the history of Atlanta's Continuum of Care, limited governmental funding, and a reliance on non-governmental actors as both providers and funders. The state and economic elite policy initiatives remain separate and constrain decision-making and policy implementation as a result, while the institutional arrangements of Atlanta as a metropolitan area have direct, negative effects on all policy efforts and any policy coordination overall. In summary, the limited coordination between interests governing homeless policy reduces the implementation of publicly funded policy alternatives for Atlanta and increases the policy alternatives for privately pursued, reactionary policies.

Chapter 7 presents the case study results from Shreveport. Unlike San Francisco and Atlanta, Shreveport serves as the representative case for municipalities without a local government level supportive housing policy (see Chapter 3). Shreveport is a case where the Continuum of Care and municipal policy goals, decision-making, and implementation remain very separate. The separation is evident in policy decision-making and implementation, where the municipality has little to no involvement in homeless policy aside from coordinating passthrough federal funding. The Continuum of Care operates independently, debating homeless policy choices and implementing policies without aid and little to no input from the local government. The lack of involvement by Shreveport's municipal government presents direct barriers to supportive housing policy design and implementation in Shreveport by restricting the authority and the resources available to the Continuum of Care to coordinate policy activities.

Unlike Atlanta and San Francisco, where the local government and the Continuum of Care have merged to jointly govern homeless policy, the Shreveport Continuum of Care remains independent, which effectively constrains their ability to design and implement some policy changes. As discussed in the chapter, policing remains a persistent challenge in interactions with persons experiencing chronic homelessness, as well as a challenge for federal requirements to move away from policing responses to homelessness and chronic homelessness. Since the Continuum of Care has no municipal authority, they are limited in their ability to coordinate with the Shreveport Police Department, to require trainings on best practices or responses to individuals experiencing chronic homelessness and severe mental illness, or to support coordinated entry practices with the assistance of police officers. Zoning remains another challenge. With limited ability to participate in municipal debates, the Continuum of Care is often disadvantaged in debates over new shelter or low-income housing constructions and is often overshadowed by economic elites in the Downtown Development Authority. This is a stark comparison to San Francisco, and even Atlanta, where Continuum of Care actors are a part of the municipal bureaucracy, are heavily involved in policy design with city officials, and are able to coordinate with and facilitate design and implementation of policing interventions, supportive housing policy design and development, and municipal-level funding initiatives. In Shreveport's case, the complete decentralization promotes policy opportunities for private actors and inhibits policy opportunities for the publicly funded Continuum of Care mechanisms.

Chapter 8 synthesizes the primary findings from the results of the quantitative and qualitative analysis and subsequently provides recommendations for policy makers to improve homeless policy governance systems to design and deliver policies that successfully ameliorate chronic homelessness. Overcoming the challenges associated with decentralization and policy conflict or a lack of coordination across policy interests to address chronic homelessness in municipalities across the United States will be a big hurdle requiring substantial changes. Primary recommendations for reform include, first, aligning Continuums of Care with municipal government, formally or informally, to ensure that the Continuums have access to necessary resources and governmental authority to be able to design and implement policy across the variety of policy spaces—housing, healthcare, behavioral health, policing, and incarceration. Second, improving participatory equity in homeless policy decision-making to include minority groups and persons who are currently or formerly homeless will improve policy design and implementation to ensure that policies targeting persons experiencing homelessness work to their intended goals, do not exacerbate harm to persons at risk of or experiencing homelessness, and protect policy processes from bias toward economic elite stakeholders in pluralistic settings. Lastly, I recommend steps to help align historically and contemporary tangential state-level policies that provide services for persons experiencing chronic homelessness but, by virtue of not being *designed* to target chronic homelessness, fail in policy implementation by engendering barriers to local homeless policy solutions.

CHAPTER 2

Homeless Politics in the United States

Theories of the Ungoverned and Unwanted

Public health as a discipline studies issues influenced by local politics and policies that are primarily implemented and, in many cases, governed by county level public health departments. Yet the world of public health policy tends to focus on the politics and policies at the state and federal level. Obscuring the role of local politics and in designing and implementing public health policies inaccurately portrays the functioning of public health systems and can lead to incorrect or incomplete assumptions about the effects of health politics on public health outcomes. Homelessness is no exception. Homelessness is a policy space with a long history of expanded governing authority for local governments and communities. To understand policy outcomes in homelessness governance, we must draw from the theories of urban politics and intergovernmental relations that have been developed to explain social policy.

In this chapter, I outline a theory illustrating how limited coordination between fragmented policy interests—local governments, Continuums of Care, local elites, and states—and strong trend in decentralization in homeless policy governance interact to diminish policy opportunities for publicly funded, evidence-based supportive housing policy at the municipal level and subsequently increase policy opportunities for private actors. The separation and conflict between these fragmented policy spaces end in increased challenges to establishing and implementing effective policy solutions to end chronic homelessness. Constraints include limited

Ungoverned and Out of Sight. Charley E. Willison, Oxford University Press (2021). © Oxford University Press.
DOI: 10.1093/oso/9780197548325.003.0002

involvement by municipal governments in many cases, which may restrict supportive housing policy due to inherent funding limitations and service coordination; inequity in political participation that generally excludes at-risk populations or bias participation in favor of economic elites in pluralistic political environments; and, finally, relatively absent state level support and misalignment of existing, tangential state level policies that contribute to resource constraints for local actors and may create administrative burdens due to misaligned policy goals.

I first outline the history of municipal governance in social service and health policy and compare that to the decentralized and delegated development of homeless policy governance from its inception in the 1980s. I then review literature on the delegated state in social and health policy to consider the implications of formal, delegated state governance for homeless policy mechanisms in practice in pluralistic municipal political systems. Here, I specifically consider the role of local economic elites and municipal institutions and consider their interactions with delegated systems to explore mechanisms of policy functioning in local homeless policy. Lastly, I review the existing literature on social construction in health and social services policy to explore what motivates different local actors to pursue different policies to address chronic homelessness. I combine these insights on decentralization and the delegated state, political participation, and social construction to outline my new theory of homeless policy politics.

INTERGOVERNMENTAL RELATIONS AND LOCAL POLITICS IN PUBLIC HEALTH AND HOMELESS POLICY

Most public health literature does not examine the role of local governments. The literature is mainly restricted to discussions of community health. The political structure and, foremost, the importance of local governments in designing and implementing many public health services are almost entirely absent from public health rhetoric. Discussions are usually directed to the relationship between local and state public health agencies, with local public health agencies seen as responsive to state wishes. In reality, a large division of public health depends on local decision-making. And in the case of chronic homelessness, states are typically bypassed, and most decision-making governing the direction of homeless governance takes place directly between cities and the federal government.

Most public health and political science literature exploring public policy decision-making concerns state and federal units. There is limited academic work on federal–local relations (Davidson 2007). This is perhaps because cities are not recognized as legitimate, independent entities under the constitution (Bowers 2015, 11). The constitution describes only two levels of government: the federal government and the states (Ross and Levine 2001a). The constitution prescribes any governmental authority given to cities must be conferred to the local government by the state (Ross and Levine 2001a). In 1868, an Iowa Supreme Court ruling preserved the dependent status of cities (J. F. Dillon 1911). The ruling, known as Dillon's Rule, labeled cities as "creatures of the state," possessing only those powers delegated to them by the states. The ruling described cities as "municipal corporations," whose governance powers may be brought forth, amended, or destroyed by state government as it sees fit (J. F. Dillon 1911). Dillon's Rule also established the concept of preemption. Preemption is the rule denoting state precedence over local governments in policymaking (Berman 1997). States can supersede local actions and deny local government authority. In public health policy, preemption plays an important role in shaping state public health policy, from gun control to tobacco control (Berman 1997). Today, Dillon's Rule remains the dominant doctrine of municipal law, shaping authority granted to cities and the way that cities' roles are perceived in intergovernmental relations (Ross and Levine 2001a).

Yet, this narrow conception of federalism obscures a key piece of public policy decision-making relations. Cities play a large role in establishing and implementing public policies that shape local economics and population health (Davidson 2007, 960; Sellers 2002). Furthermore, federal–local relations have played a significant role in establishing municipal priorities, policies, and initiatives (Davidson 2007; Elazar 1991). In many policy cases, cities are not dependent on states and often have more power as political actors and strong relationships with the federal government (Davidson 2007; Miller 2002; Shipan 2006). The federalism literature and history describes the current state of intergovernmental relations as much more of an amalgamation of authority, rather than a clear-cut hierarchy determining roles and responsibilities (Ross and Levine 2001b). As interpretations and statutes of federalism evolved, cities preserved and acquired a great deal of discretion to determine the shape and effects of federal programs in their jurisdiction (Ross and Levine 2001b).

Cooperative federalism, or "marble cake" federalism, first emerged under Roosevelt during the Great Depression and the New Deal, establishing cooperation between national and subnational governments to deal with domestic policy problems (Glendening and Reeves 1984). Local agencies and officials, as opposed to states, were charged with implementing the new federally funded social programs (Ross and Levine 2001b). This was a sharp contrast from "old-style" federalism, or the constitutional interpretation as previously discussed that focused on Supreme Court interpretations of the constitution regarding which powers belong to which level of government, focusing on the relationship between the states and the federal government (Ross and Levine 2001b). The role of cities in implementing federal policy initiatives grew from the New Deal, and expanded under World War II through the 1960s under Lyndon Johnson's Great Society (Ross and Levine 2001b). The programs fostered strong federal–city connections, increasing the prominence of cities in the intergovernmental system (D. B. Walker 1995). These relationships resulted in *direct federalism*, a system based on federal–city relationships that circumvented states (Ross and Levine 2001b; D. B. Walker 1995). Direct federalism and strong city prominence continued through the 1970s. This relationship changed in the 1980s, when funding for federal social programs was cut substantially (Johnson 1991; Weicher 1984; Weir, Orloff, and Skocpol 1988). The federal government devolved authority and responsibility for social programs to cities and markedly limited federal financial support (Conlan 1998). Despite this shift, the long precedence through the 20th century for direct federalism, during which many core U.S. health policies and programs were established, highlights the importance of evaluating the effects of intergovernmental relations on public health policy outcomes, as opposed to focusing solely on constitutional federalism (Glendening and Reeves 1984; D. B. Walker 1995).

While existing scholarship has generally neglected the important role of direct federalism in health policy decision-making and implementation, which this research will emphasize, existing scholarship has also overlooked the often lateral relationship between existing state-level policies and local efforts in policy spaces that are primarily governed by municipal actors. For example, much health policy scholarship on the relationship between homelessness and Medicaid neglects to recognize or examine the fact that homeless policy is not governed at the state level (Bharel et al. 2013; Cassidy 2016; Dipietro, Artiga, and Gates 2014; Rinker 2019; Tsai et al. 2013; Warfield, Dipietro, and Artiga 2016). Therefore, when much of this scholarship seeks to explore the effects of Medicaid policy on homelessness, the mechanisms are often invalid, and we receive an incomplete understanding of the policy processes at work and why Medicaid may or may not be working well for persons experiencing homelessness. By designing and providing accurate measures of homeless policy governance, this research adds great value to existing scholarship on the relationships between state level policies and homelessness.

Neoliberalism and the Submerged State

Where health politics often leaves municipalities out of the picture, there has been a lot of research on the role of neoliberalism and the implications of delegating social services in health and welfare policy to nongovernmental actors across levels of government. I attempt to connect the literature on health politics and federalism with scholarship on the delegated welfare state by linking the influence of neoliberalism on municipal policy to changes in public health service programming, of which homelessness is a key issue. Neoliberalism and the growth of the delegated state explains the shift to municipalities and communities to alone shoulder the burdens of managing homelessness and behavioral health in the mid-late 20th century when they would have historically received federal aid to assist their efforts, providing key historical context to understand today's governance arrangements for homeless services. This scholarship also leads into the strategic role of social construction in promoting neoliberal social policies. My research provides a contemporary understanding of this historical phenomenon by demonstrating the persistent role of social construction in homeless policy today and how social construction interacts with delegated governance.

Neoliberalism was a political platform pushed most notably in the 1980s by Reagan in the United States and Thatcher in the United Kingdom, which forever shaped the U.S. welfare state (Cole 2006; K. Jacobs and Manzi 2013; Johnson 1991; Lamb and Twombly 1993). Neoliberalism is defined by a platform of governmental decentralization coupled with promoting private business partnerships with local governments as a means of further decentralizing and delegating responsibility (K. Jacobs and Manzi 2013).

The decentralization of responsibility to nongovernmental actors in the 1980s was a strategic move by conservative political actors. There were two primary goals of decentralization. The first, was to align with traditional conservative notions of government by reducing the size of government and therefore leaving more room for private business growth (Soss, Fording, and Schram 2011). Yet the second goal, less often discussed, was the primary impetus for decentralization and specifically the growth of the delegated state. That was the goal to undercut and demobilize liberal stakeholder coalitions that arose from the social rights movements—women's rights, racial/ethnic minority rights, healthcare, the elderly, and disability rights. The social rights movements had successfully coalesced around these issues to establish major legislation and expansion of government services and programming, including Medicare and Medicaid, the Voting Rights Act, *Roe v. Wade*, etc. Conservatives were increasingly threatened. In response to major liberal successes, conservative actors found a way to demobilize liberal actors by cutting social service programming and therefore shifting interest group coalitions away from activism to direct service providers roles to fill the social service gap (Luker 1996; Skocpol and Pierson 2007; Soss, Fording, and Schram 2011; Weaver 2007). As a result, conservative actors were able to diminish liberal activist coalitions and maintain some sort of private social service provision, while promoting the illusion that the government is not involved (Diiulio 2012; Soss, Fording, and Schram 2011).

At the same time as the strategic demobilization of the activist state during the civil rights movement, another movement was happening in behavioral healthcare. Across industrialized nations, national campaigns and legislation were promoted to close public psychiatric institutions, in response to their history of abuse and neglect for persons with serious mental illness. This phenomenon of deinstitutionalization was intended to be followed up with alternate care models for persons with serious mental health needs (Goldman and Morrissey 1985; Shadish 1984). In the United States, the intention was to create models of community care, where persons would receive targeted outpatient care directed by their communities or delegated to nongovernmental organizations. However, the legislation that would have paid for community behavioral healthcare models was never implemented (Grob 1994; Morrissey and Goldman 1984; Sisti, Segal, and Emanuel 2015). As a result, care for serious mental illness in the United States was actively devolved and demobilized by failing to re-establish necessary behavioral healthcare capacity. When homelessness arose as a policy problem in the 1980s, existing infrastructure to manage homelessness had been cut and shifted back to communities of nongovernmental actors, setting the state for today's complex system of delegation and limited governmental participation.

The decentralization of responsibility and the increasing absence of federal funding for social services under Reagan and following deinstitutionalization led to the development of the "submerged" or "delegated" state as a primary mechanism for delivering housing and supportive medical and behavioral health services for the homeless and many other welfare programs (Dreier 2007; K. Jacobs and Manzi 2013; Lamb and Twombly 1993). The emerging delegated state marked an important change in intergovernmental relations, where communities—and not just local governments but specifically local, nongovernmental actors—came to play vital roles in designing and delivering social policy (Diiulio 2012), including homelessness policy and programming.

The delegated state is defined as a set of "invisible," or indirect, mechanisms guiding governmental activities and programs for the public through nongovernmental organizations, such as private for-profit and nonprofit organizations (Hackett 2017). These invisible mechanisms include governments incentivizing private activity or delivery of certain social services by giving subsidies or benefits to the private organizations via tax subsidies, rebates, and credits (Hackett 2017; Mettler 2011; Morgan and Campbell 2011). An example of the submerged state at work is providing private companies with tax breaks and subsidies to provide low-income housing (Hackett 2017; Willison 2017). Governments are then indirectly paying for public programs, without actually delivering the programs themselves.

One challenge with incentivizing submerged state activity is that it unintentionally created a new constituency of stakeholders. This new constituency takes the form of persons who receive services from delegated state actors and persons who are employed in the delegated state as workers at community-based organizations. This makes reining in submerged state spending *or* recentralization very challenging, as this new host of constituents rely on the submerged state for social service delivery and delegated state actors rely on its existence for their livelihoods. Therefore, the growth of the submerged state, while promoting the importance of cities as key decision makers, is described as actually undermining local *governmental* authority for delivering these services, due to this new policy conflict between local governments and competing private sector interests (Cole 2006; Kemp 2007, 113; Letelier 2005; Jacobs and Manzi 2013).

Although the growth of the delegated state increased the separation of municipal government and delegated state authority in U.S. homeless policy, there are other instances where the growth of the delegated state may alleviate intergovernmental conflict. In cases where there are high levels of policy conflict between levels of government or within one level of government, the submerged state can and historically has filled important service gaps. Submerged state actors—for example, nonprofit organizations delivering medical services, housing, and other basic needs services—are critical participants in homeless programming and may fill these service needs during times of government conflict or service reduction (Willison 2017). As discussed, the entire federal system governing homeless service delivery relies on participation from submerged state actors. Although the delegated state can mechanistically reduce conflict—for example, when states and localities disagree by filling service gaps—the institutional arrangements between municipalities and the delegated state can cause conflict by perpetuating separate policy systems. Conflict may arise here when those isolated, delegated systems restrict flow of essential resources and services to allow for effective policy design and implementation such as regulatory powers and funding.

This strategic federal decentralization enshrined the precedence for municipalities—specifically, municipalities as *communities* in their partnerships with local nongovernmental organizations—as the primary entities responsible for designing and delivering housing and supportive behavioral and health services to the homeless (Johnson 1991; Lamb and Twombly 1993; Morrissey and Goldman 1984). In homelessness policy, this took the form of establishing designated federal funding for homelessness to be awarded to municipally concentrated groups of nongovernmental actors, or the Continuums of Care.

In effect, the policy histories of delegating responsibility for homelessness to locally organized nongovernmental actors created strong incentives to limit municipal governmental involvement. Nongovernmental organizations have been providing services to mitigate homelessness since the 1980s and have been formally organized as the Continuums of Care since the 1990s (U.S. Department of Housing and Urban Development 2012). These organizations have a desire to persist to serve their communities and remain as employers for many social service providers (Diiulio 2012). With well-organized stakeholder coalitions and service provider networks for homelessness programming, local governments face limited incentives to step into homelessness governance. In 2014, local governments were only involved in 38% of the Continuums of Care across the United States (Jarpe, Mosely, and Smith 2019). Many local governments face revenue constraints and budget shortfalls that may further disincentivize participation in additional governing activities. Overall, neoliberalism and the resulting decentralization of homelessness governance has led to a persistent separation between municipal governments and the Continuums of Care. These nongovernmental actors shoulder the responsibility of designing and delivering solutions to homelessness across the United States. As this research will show, this delegation creates a fragmented policy space where actors responsible for homeless policy may not have access to necessary resources by virtue of complete decentralization, and policy conflict often arises between local governments and the Continuums of Care.

Now that we understand how homeless policy developed in the United States—in particular, the strategic decentralization and delegation of homeless policy governance creating fragmented municipal and Continuum of Care systems—we need to look at what previous research tells us about the implications of this governing arrangement for homeless policy. Do we know if it worked? Did it create challenges? This section considers how increased policy conflict resulting from neoliberalism and submerged state growth brought new challenges for local homelessness policy design and implementation. This literature provides insight into understanding the persistence of local authority in the case of homeless policy by examining: which actors have authority; how that authority is distributed; and how the distribution of authority affects decision-making by determining who can and cannot participate in policy-making and how economic interests interact with authority and plurality in participation.

A paradox of submerged state actors is that their services are voluntary. Providing programming and service delivery is not mandated, although actors receive federal funding and incentives for doing the work. Starting in 1995, if local actors want to receive federal funding to address homelessness, they must have established a Continuum of Care (as the organization that will receive federal funding, design programming, and distribute the funding to other local actors to deliver services; US Department of Housing and Urban Development 2012, 3). Yet, local action to mitigate homelessness is not mandated by the federal government. This is completely voluntary. Further, although the federal government has established rules governing how federal funding must be used by Continuum of Cares, the Continuum of Cares have primary authority to decide how they use funding, what to prioritize, and how to implement homelessness programming (Jarpe, Mosely, and Smith 2019; Lee and McGuire 2017). This strong deference to the delegated state in homelessness policy is a benefit when governments may otherwise be absent, but it is a cost when the voluntary nature of homeless policy may lead to effective or ineffective heterogeneity in services design and delivery (Weir and Schirmer 2018).

Beyond local variation in the establishment and delivery of homeless services, deference to the delegated state becomes voluntary by means of authority. Complete delegation of homelessness governance to nongovernmental actors generates a policy space where regulations governing the Continuum of Care may not implemented as a result of the limited to no authority Continuum of Care actors have over any municipal services, or other private or nongovernmental actors, to coordinate policy implementation effectively. Continuum of Cares in this space can only ask and hope for buy-in from critical actors. In cases where actors governing housing resources, zoning and building permitting, police activity, and even county or parish level health insurance enrollment choose not to participate, homelessness policy and programming may fail or stagnate with serious consequences for persons experiencing homelessness and local economies (Willison 2017). As previously discussed, other scholarship has demonstrated the challenges associated with institutional devolution and delegation in education and housing policy (Cronley 2010; Hackett 2017; Johnson 1991), yet the influence of delegated authority on homeless policy has hardly been evaluated (National Academies of Sciences Engineering and Medicine 2018, 105–107). This book seeks to fill that gap. Without any real governing authority for the majority of Continuum of Cares in the United States, homelessness policy under the delegated state remains voluntary. In public health, a similar scenario would be delegating vaccine policy to locally arranged groups of community-based organizations.

How decision-making authority is dispersed between governmental and nongovernmental actors also has to do a lot with the need for policy capacity and the potential for policy conflict. Existing health politics research on policy capacity tells us a lot about the importance of policy capacity in general and in delegated contexts specifically. Policy capacity is the part of government that turns ideas into workable, well-designed policies able to succeed in their designated context (Greer, Wismar, and Figuera, 2016; Page 2006). Policy capacity relies on governments consulting or positioning policy experts to design policies tailored to work in the designated context and for desired outcome(s). Naturally, many of these actors are members of the delegated state. Policy capacity matters in homeless policy because public authorities may not understand all of the consequences of various homelessness strategies and therefore be unable to make policy decisions that deliver the intended policy goals (Lieberherr, Maarse, and Jeurissen 2016). However, for policies to be successful and achieve to the desired goals, the policy must also be aligned with available resources (Greer et al. 2016, 39–40). Aligning policies with available resources becomes increasingly challenging in complex and contentious political environments. Decentralization may make resource allocation among nongovernmental actors more challenging, as delegated state actors may have more difficulty acquiring and retaining funding than governmental actors (Mettler 2016; Weir and Schirmer 2018).

However, policy capacity may also conflict with political interests. Policy makers rely on external expertise to design policy, and regulatory expertise is strongly correlated with adopting evidence-based policies (Bruff 2010;

Fischer 2009; Greer et al. 2016, 40). Yet, increasing policy capacity does not guarantee improved policy design or implementation, due to potential conflict in policy preferences between embedded experts, politicians, and other stakeholders (Gailmard and Patty 2007). This may lead to two outcomes. Politicians may recognize expertise, especially if it aligns with their own policy preferences, but may face opposition from other constituent groups (Huber and Shipan 2002). If politicians do not agree with expertise and/or if expertise is not aligned with their policy preferences, politicians may seek to reduce or decentralize policy capacity or delay policy implementation.

This book expands existing research on policy capacity in health politics and applies it to homeless policy in the interaction between delegation and policy efficacy. In homeless policy today, this conflict is very apparent. Local governments in many cases have adopted both harmful policing strategies *and* evidence-based supportive housing policies, (Nacgourney 2016; D. Smith 2016) in response to competing interests between municipal economic elites and stakeholders promoting evidence based policies (such as behavioral health providers and the Continuums of Care). Policy conflict arising from policy capacity may result in a further separation of municipal government and the Continuums of Care. If the Continuum of Cares have relatively strong policy capacity but no role in municipal government and elected officials' preferences conflict with Continuum of Care initiatives, municipalities may be further disincentivized to participate in homeless policy and may be directly incentivized to utilize competing policies in the form of policing.

Existing research on municipal fragmentation can also tell us a lot about when and why there may be more or less policy conflict in a specific policy arena. Fragmentation refers to the number of municipal governments in a county area (Berry 2009; Goodman 2015). Municipal fragmentation is a unique issue that may unintentionally introduce more policy conflict into municipal policy debates. Municipal fragmentation affects the ability of different stakeholders to participate in political decision-making and the ability for actors to coordinate policy approaches successfully or even develop coordinated approaches in the first place. Municipal incorporation was a popular phenomenon in the 20th century, where pockets of economic elites would establish their own local governments in an attempt to evade city property taxes and have more concentrated control over public goods like schools and libraries (Hogen-Esch 2011). However, such incorporation often maintained relationships with the primary municipality for services such as water, garbage disposal, and police and fire services (Hogen-Esch 2011; Peterson 1981; Ross and Levine 2001b). The result of fragmentation was an increasing disjuncture of centralized municipal services and decision-making (Frederickson 1999).

Homeless policies (in fully delegated arrangements and centralized municipal policy arrangements) are often intergovernmental policies pursued by city and county governments. These intergovernmental policies therefore require buy-in and action from multiple departments across multiple jurisdictions and municipal services. Increased municipal fragmentation may act as a barrier to establishing supportive housing policy approaches by preventing necessary policy coordination between relevant jurisdictions and services and concentrating relevant stakeholder power in certain jurisdictions over others. While fragmentation is a common concern in urban politics literature, the implications of municipal fragmentation are almost never explored in public health scholarship, and micropolitan analyses focus on downstream characteristics of jurisdictional arrangements, such as segregation and neighborhood characteristics (Chetty, Hendren, and Katz 2015; Cook et al. 2017; Fenelon et al. 2017; Rauh, Landrigan, and Claudio 2008). While this research identifies important health inequities, this omitted variable bias, excluding upstream, institutional arrangements that engender the disparate neighborhood characteristics, may constrain our understanding of the causes of these adverse health outcomes in the first place. This research expands the current scholarship by examining municipal fragmentation as a relevant factor in public health policy outcomes. Further, existing scholarship on fragmentation does not consider the role of the delegated state. This book argues that delegation and fragmentation may interact to increase barriers to supportive housing policy by further restricting authority and coordination between relevant governance systems.

Finally, actors' ability to participate in political debates and decision-making is affected by the political institutional structures in place. Whether or not local stakeholders participate in politics matters because their participation affects the policy decision-making process, which affects the outcome of interest—what homeless policies municipalities pursue (Lillvis and Greer 2016). Elite stakeholders' political participation may be restricted or enhanced depending on system rules (Mickey 2008, 11). Even economic elites, such as real estate companies, may not necessarily be able to translate their economic power into political power depending on the political institutional structures that allow for greater or less public participation (Mickey 2008). This works both ways—either pushing toward or away from supportive housing depending on the preferences of the participating actors. However, in more pluralistic systems, economic power generally translates into political influence (Einstein, Palmer, and Glick 2018; Mickey 2015; Trounstine 2008; Zannoni 1978).

In homeless policy, economic elites are typically opposed to supportive housing initiatives, regardless of ideology (Kim 2000; Piat 2000; Sisco 2017). Economic elites, in the context of homeless policy, may include organized, corporate interests, such as Downtown Development Associations, housing corporations, or other entities with vested interest in municipal property such as movie productions and sports (Gustafson 2013). By contrast, economic elites may also include groups, formally or informally organized, of wealthy homeowners (Einstein, Palmer, and Glick 2018; Takahashi 1997; Trounstine 2020). Because of this opposition to supportive housing policy, degrees of plurality in debates over homeless policy may matter significantly for homeless policy outcomes. For example, in municipalities with more pluralistic systems, economic elites may obscure minority groups' preferences including persons at risk of or who are formerly or currently homeless, the majority of whom are racial/ethnic minority group members. Thus, the preferences of political-economic elites matter greatly in these systems in terms of the outcomes for city decision-making. My research expands existing local political economy research by linking the influence of delegated state arrangements, policy capacity, municipal fragmentation, and political participation to understand more fully the complex policy mechanisms facing homeless policy development and implementation.

SOCIAL CONSTRUCTION—WHEN POLICING RESPONSES CONFLICT WITH PUBLIC HEALTH

As discussed in the Chapter 1 of this volume, the Continuums of Care since 2015 have been required by federal funding to move toward adopting supportive housing with a Housing First approach as their primary means to addressing homelessness (Goodloe 2015). At the same time, federal funding requirements now also expect the Continuums of Care to reduce *criminalization* of homelessness, or punitive law enforcement or policing responses to individuals experiencing chronic homelessness (T. Bauman et al. 2017; Tars 2015).[1] Criminalization responses directly conflict with supportive housing policy goals and implementation, by addressing behaviors associated with homelessness instead of the causes of homelessness. This generally includes "quality of life" laws, such as eating, sitting down, and sleeping in public spaces, which are almost entirely applied to persons experiencing homelessness rather than members of the public, broadly speaking (Robinson 2019). Criminalization responses are implemented or enforced through local policing, arresting, citing, or removing persons experiencing homelessness and/or their possessions from public spaces. These reactive policing responses to chronic homelessness ultimately redirect individuals into the criminal justice system as opposed to health and social services, leading to ongoing cycles of incarceration and homelessness, most notoriously among persons experiencing chronic homelessness (Berkeley Law Policy Advocacy Clinic 2018; Hawthorne et al. 2012; Segal, Frasso, and Sisti 2018).

Extensive research has examined the effects of criminalization on health outcomes, economic outcomes, and political indicators, and other research has documented, described, and defined criminalization of racial/ethnic minority groups in other policy areas. There is less research considering the politics of criminalization or the political challenges associated with reforming ineffective criminalization policies. Furthermore, there is even less research analyzing effects of the political institutional relationship and the federated division of authority on local political decision-making related to criminalization of at-risk or oppressed groups. There is also a greater need for understanding and grounding how social constructions of target populations play into the greater political decision-making environment and intergovernmental relations. This research expands this literature by exploring the political processes involved in criminalization, the relationship between social construction and criminalization, and the effects of historically institutionalized criminalization on current political decision-making to better understand municipal homeless policy outcomes.

The social construction of a target population refers to "the recognition of the shared characteristics that distinguish a target population as socially meaningful, and the attribution of specific, valence-oriented values, symbols, and images to the characteristics" (Schneider and Ingram 1993). Social constructions are stereotypes of certain populations of people created by socialization, politics, culture, history, etc. Social construction can be positive or negative. Positive constructions include impressions such as "deserving," "well-meaning," "intelligent," etc. Negative constructions often include "violent," "undeserving," "criminal," and "lazy" (Schneider and Ingram 1993).

Schneider and Ingram's (1993) theory of the social construction of target populations contends that social constructions influence policy agenda-setting, selection of policy tools, and the rationales that legitimize policy choices. Schneider and Ingram see social construction as implicit biases that become engrained in policy by affecting the way certain policy makers and constituents are oriented to different groups. The theory made a great contribution to political science because it offered an additional explanation for why some groups are prioritized more than others in social policy. Thus, this theory proposes that in such contexts, as in this case, at-risk populations may be criminalized based on stereotypes and misconceptions as a means of solving a problem in the eyes of wider society (Clifford and Piston 2017; Perez, Leifman, and Estrada 2003; Sisco 2017). However, much of this literature lacks an overarching or synthesized explanation of how social constructions work in conjunction with other political structures, incentives, and tools to explain policy decision-making more completely. This book seeks to integrate existing theory on social construction to generate a more complete theory about the interaction between social construction and existing political structures and how social construction may be leveraged as a strategic political tool by well-positioned actors in pluralistic systems.

History of Criminalization

Criminalization as a social policy approach occurred across various contexts throughout the history of the United States and continues today. People who are chronically homeless and individuals who are significantly more likely to be homeless as a result of an untreated mental health or substance use disorder have historically been associated with criminal deviancy, derangement, and violence (Brescia 2015; Cooper 2013; Mulvey and White 2013; Perez, Leifman, and Estrada 2003; Saks 2013). The first waves of homeless persons in the United States were primarily single men, known colloquially as "tramps" and "thieves" in the late 19th century (Grob 1994). The connection to mental health was not suggested until the growth of psychiatry in the turn of the century, although the etiology of psychosis was not understood for much longer (Grob 1994). Such conceptions of derangement erupted in the early 20th century with the rise of psychiatry; the growth of psychiatric institutions, or "insane asylums"; and insanity in media (Eisenberg 1988). These notions persisted after deinstitutionalization (see previous discussion) in the 1960s as myths ascended asserting that the majority of the homeless were either psychotic or deranged alcoholics and drug abusers (Grob 1994; Jones 2015).

Most of the literature evaluating criminalization in social policy focuses on two aspects. First, criminalization came to social policy through social construction and stigmatization. Here, a moral weight is associated with certain perceived individual or group characteristics, which serve to rationalize punitive responses to such characteristics. Second, criminalization is often utilized as a purposeful political or economic tool. Criminalization here leverages social constructions of targeted populations to achieve desired economic or political ends.

Moral and Political Criminalization—Deviancy and Disenfranchisement

Empirical evidence shows homelessness results from structural problems at a societal level. This includes insufficient income and lack of affordable housing, domestic violence, unemployment, poverty, mental illness and the lack of critical services, and substance abuse and the lack of needed services (National Academies of Sciences Engineering and Medicine 2018; National Law Center on Homelessness and Poverty 2015; U.S. Interagency Council on Homelessness 2015). These factors include the converging relationship between individual and structural factors. Despite this knowledge, social policy debates persist about the roots of homelessness as a consequence of socially constructed notions of individual failures and choices (Cronley 2010).

In the United States, two main paradigms shape the debate about the causes of homelessness. The two main interpretations of the causes of homelessness are (1) individual and (2) structural interpretations. Individual interpretations suggest homelessness is a product of personal deficits, such as substance abuse, lack of personal motivation, and social isolation. Structural interpretations uphold that homelessness results from systemic factors including lack of affordable housing, employment opportunities, and lack of necessary medical and behavioral health services, aligning with empirical evidence outlining the primary causes of homelessness (Cronley 2010).

Political science research has found that elected policy makers more often attribute causes of homelessness to the individual paradigm (Clifford and Piston 2017; J. D. Wright, Rubin, and Devine 1998). Elected policy makers may be more likely to adhere to this paradigm as a result of the interaction between social construction and limited policy area expertise, as well as pressure from private industries and coalitions of elites who most often oppose structural solutions to homelessness because this position favors their short-term economic and political goals (e.g., tourism; housing development; neighborhood homogeneity, expressed as "not in my back yard," or NIMBYISM). Elected officials' limited policy area expertise may be worse in the majority of cases with no municipal government involvement in Continuum of Care activity.

In the case of elected official's interactions with economic elites, U.S. history is rife with instances of economic elites strategically utilizing negative social constructions as political tools to favor their own economic or political ends. This includes employing racist constructions of Black Americans to protect authoritarian enclaves in southern states during the civil rights movement and urban regimes of the early 20th century retaining political power through targeted campaigns of racial animus and resentment toward opposition groups (Bridges 1999; Lublin 2004; Mickey 2008, 11; 2015; Trounstine 2008). Thus, opposition to structural solutions to homelessness may arise from perverse incentives by politicians and economic elites seeking to protect their own electoral and fiscal interests. When politicians and economic elites oppose structural solutions, they may be more likely to favor short-term, criminalization responses through policing that address behaviors associated with homelessness. Ultimately, municipal elected officials today may strategically employ negative social constructions of homelessness to disincentivize supportive housing efforts and retain political support from elite coalitions.

This literature leaves open the possibility that city choices to criminalize may be the first choice of many municipalities. Criminalizing homelessness through policing as an alternative policy process to supportive housing may be perfectly rational in individual municipal contexts because people experiencing homelessness are perceived as criminal, deviant, or a nuisance, as a result of norms and social construction. Therefore, criminalization becomes the natural choice, and the alternative option to provide housing and supportive health services seems irrational.

FRAGMENTED AND COMPETING POLICY PROCESSES

Scholarship on intergovernmental relations, local political economy, and social construction are useful in explaining local decision-making in homelessness policy. Overall, these theories tell us that (1) there is a long history of municipal governance in social policy in the United States; (2) homeless policy has remained separate from this history of municipal governance and has instead had a long history of governance through delegated systems to nongovernmental actors; (3) the political power of economic elites may obscure minority group or at-risk target population preferences in highly pluralistic municipal systems; and (4) negative social constructions of homelessness are often enlisted by economic elites and elected officials to justify their own economic and electoral preferences, and these actors may oppose bureaucratic expertise when it does not align with their interests.

Yet, in short, previous research has missed several crucial components of the politics of homeless policy. Public health research has failed to consider governing structures of homeless policy, both in the context of state policies affecting homelessness and chronic homelessness and in urban health research. Moreover, the implications of an entirely delegated governance system—and how that delegated governance interacts with existing, critical elements of policy making including policy capacity, jurisdictional institutional arrangements, and political participation—have not been explored in homeless policy politics, in public health, or in political science. Finally, how people who are formerly, currently, or at-risk of homelessness are *perceived* has not been evaluated in the context of policy-making processes for homeless policy. In general, homeless policy and politics take place in a highly complex, fragmented space that we know very little about in terms of the policy space itself, how it is organized, and who participates.

COMPETING POLICY PROCESSES AND INTERESTS

I propose a theory of fragmented and competing policy processes in U.S. homeless policy governance. The theory I propose argues that (1) limited coordination between interests governing homeless policy and (2) strong trends of decentralization in homeless policy governance contribute to fewer public policy alternatives for solutions to chronic homelessness and increase the policy alternatives for private actors. Homelessness is a unique case of a health issue that is governed by an almost entirely decentralized, or delegated, nongovernmental system—both historically and today. The history of devolution and decentralization in homeless policy governance makes it a unique policy space where various actors compete and implement very different types of policies that all attempt to manage homelessness and chronic homelessness to different ends.

This book argues that homeless policy—specifically policies seeking solutions to patterns of chronic homelessness—are governed by four separate and distinct policy interests: state government, local government, local economic elites, and homeless service providers or the formal governing structure for homelessness outlined by federal policy known as the Continuums of Care. The separation and conflict between these policy interests result in increased challenges to establishing and implementing effective policy solutions to end chronic homelessness. Challenges include limited state-level support such as financial resources and/or administrative burdens due to misaligned policy goals; inequity in political participation that may exclude at-risk populations or bias participation in favor of economic elites; and, finally, limited involvement by municipal governments in many cases, which may constrain homeless programming due to inherent funding limitations and service coordination barriers.

Fully decentralized homeless policy governance to nongovernmental actors in the Continuum of Care inherently restricts actors in their ability to design and carry out policy goals as a result of institutionally constrained policy coordination, authority, and access to crucial policy resources. This includes intergovernmental relations, or the ability to coordinate with municipal governments and state governments. Coordination with states may prove inherently challenging as a result of states' historically limited role in homeless policy governance and may therefore be intensified in fully delegated arrangements of municipal homeless governance. Existing policy capacity and other jurisdictional arrangements such as municipal fragmentation may further shape delegated actor's starting point in their ability to coordinate in this already restricted environment.

When publicly funded municipal policy processes fail as a result of fragmented or uncoordinated policy approaches, economic elites or coalitions of private actors and wealthy individuals, who already often have more political power in pluralistic environments, have more leverage to enact policy goals that align with their preferences. Here, economic elites' goals, often aligned with the individual explanation of chronic homelessness, conflict with the policy goals of publicly funded supportive housing efforts. Therefore, when elites pursue short-term, reactive (and generally criminalizing) policing policies targeting homeless behaviors, they contribute to the already fragmented policy space with a policy approach that further exacerbates existing challenges to municipal supportive housing policy. By comparison, even when publicly funded policy processes succeed in *design*, the policy feedback initiated by elite utilization of conflicting, punitive policies through policing still aggravates challenges to supportive housing policy in *implementation*. For example, economic elites often enlist policing to remove persons experiencing chronic homelessness, according to quality-of-life laws, from desirable neighborhoods or business districts, redirecting persons away from services and toward the carceral state (Berkeley Law Policy Advocacy Clinic 2018; Mcnamara, Crawford, and Burns 2013; Robinson 2019).

In the end, the limited coordination between these policy sectors and the strong trend in decentralization in homeless policy governance contribute to fewer public policy alternatives to address chronic homelessness and increases the policy alternatives for private actors. Table 2.1 provides an overview of these relationships, outlining how municipal supportive

Table 2.1 MUNICIPAL HOMELESS POLICY OPPORTUNITIES

Policy Fragmentation	Governance Decentralization	
	Low	High
Low	Most policy opportunities for municipal supportive housing in design and implementation	*No* formal municipal supportive housing policy but able to implement programs across sectors
High	Formal municipal supportive housing policy, but municipal policy *fails* in implementation	*No* formal municipal supportive housing policy and very hard to implement programs across sectors

housing policy opportunities may be shaped by degrees of fragmentation across policy sectors and/or degrees of decentralization in local homeless policy governance structures.

The influence of policy conflict or fragmentation and the decentralization of homeless policy (see Table 2.1) creates a fragmented and crowded policy space that promotes collective action problems and barriers to permanent supportive housing solutions and ending chronic homelessness. This outcome is not desirable for any group. Going forward, this book presents multiple sources of evidence across various types of data (see Chapter 3 of this volume for complete details on data and methodology) to illustrate a complex, uncoordinated policy space plagued by the institutional path dependence of decentralization and delegation and the social construction of homelessness in the local political economy.

CHAPTER 3

Seeking Deeper Explanations

Case Selection and Qualitative Analysis

This chapter provides an overview of the data and methods I used to conduct this research to understand why municipalities approach chronic homelessness in different ways and why municipalities may or may not employ evidence-based strategies to address chronic homelessness. This chapter describes the rationale for conducting a mixed methods, explanatory sequential design, or the use of quantitative data, to first explore trends in an understudied subject, followed by in-depth qualitative analyses to explain the mechanisms behind the broader trends. I then outline the quantitative data, sample selection, and methodological approaches. This chapter subsequently discusses the case selection strategy stemming from the results from the national analysis and the qualitative methods and data.

RESEARCH DESIGN

As discussed in the Chapter 1, this book uses a mixed methods research design to adapt to data constraints on the topic of homeless policy. Mixed methods research is particularly useful for data-constrained scenarios, because researchers are offered multiple avenues to examine a research question and gather data, as opposed to focusing on one data source that may be insufficient to interrogate the research question. This book uses a mixed methods, explanatory sequential design. This means that I begin with a quantitative approach and end with a qualitative approach. The qualitative

Ungoverned and Out of Sight. Charley E. Willison, Oxford University Press (2021). © Oxford University Press.
DOI: 10.1093/oso/9780197548325.003.0003

approach itself is directly informed by the findings from the quantitative analysis. The key aspect of this design, as mentioned, is that it is meant to be used in scenarios with little existing research or data limitations. To overcome these constraints, this research design uses available quantitative data as an initial *exploratory* quantitative component to gain critical information about the scope of the issue and relevant trends in the data. In the next phase, the qualitative, or *explanatory*, approach addresses the limitations in the quantitative data by conducting more depth analyses, directly informed by the findings from the quantitative research or expanding on these initial results to understand the mechanisms at work and the temporality. Qualitative analysis is particularly effective in policy and politics research, where causal mechanisms are very complex and interwoven, providing a more complete picture of the causal processes at work, building from the quantitative analysis.

DATA AND METHODS

A novel and comprehensive cross-sectional data set was developed to document and measure municipal supportive housing policy choices and key political factors associated with these choices (Willison 2020). There were 402 Continuums of Care, the formal governance structures for homeless policy, comprised mostly of locally organized nongovernmental actors, in the United States in 2016. Of those 402 Continuums of Care, 354 were associated with a municipal area (i.e., categorized as "municipal" Continuums of Care). The others are state or regional Continuums of Care, which were excluded from this research.

The data set I created is comprised of 232 municipalities of 354 municipal Continuum of Cares from the U.S. Department of Housing and Urban Development (HUD) 2016 Continuum of Care database to control for cities directly receiving federal homeless funding. The final sample accounts for 66% of all Continuum of Cares in the United States. Municipalities were chosen based on their inclusion in the HUD 2016 Point-in-Time count survey, therefore selecting municipalities with a Continuum of Care that is receiving federal funding for homelessness solutions (HUD 2017c). The full sample selection strategy is described in Appendix A. This research is interested in the presence of municipal-level policies since municipalities play a key role in developing, funding, and implementing Continuum of Care policies and programming.[1]

It is important to define "municipality" as measured, here. Municipalities, broadly, refer to units of local government including cities and or counties.

This research purposefully does not choose between cities and counties in this analysis but instead identifies the unit of analysis as local government jurisdictions existing within the Continuum of Care that are primarily organized at the municipal level (e.g., one Continuum of Care in one city/county unit).[2]

Outcome Variable

In 2017, municipal-level supportive housing policies were selected from the municipal codes and regulations database Municode (2020) and cross-validated against city and county websites for each municipal Continuum of Care. To collect municipal homeless policy outcomes, a total of 464 city and county websites were reviewed (the total number of governmental websites for all cities and counties associated with the 232 Continuum of Cares in the data set), in addition to over 200 municipal codes available in the Municode database. The strategy identified 243 municipal-level policies. A municipal policy was coded as "supportive housing" if a locality (city or county government) had one or more of the following: municipal plan(s), guidelines, regulations and/or statutes establishing supportive housing, permanent supportive housing, and or Housing First as the local government's approach to chronic homelessness.

Independent Variables

The complete list of variables, their measurement, and their source is described in detail in Table 3.1 and summarized here. See Appendix A for complete descriptions of variable coding for the fuzzy set qualitative comparative analysis (fsQCA) and Stata™. There were three categories of independent variables: political institutions, social construction, and control variables. Political institutions include who may participate and the way actors coordinate with each other and participate in political decision-making processes influencing municipal adoption of supportive housing policy. These comprise measures of municipal fragmentation; ideology; intergovernmental relations, including Medicaid expansion; and various interest group presence such as nonprofit healthcare providers and tourism. Political institutions matter in understanding what factors may influence decision-making toward or away from municipal participation in supportive housing policy. Social construction variables are related to perceptions of the target population (chronically homeless persons), which

Table 3.1 VARIABLES

Political Institutions	Description	Social Construction	Description	Controls	Description
Municipal fragmentation area (U.S. Census Bureau 2012a, 2012b)	Number of general governments per county; fragmentation inhibits policy coordination (Berry 2009; Hogen-Esch 2011)	Percentage Black (U.S. Census Bureau 2017)	Social construction of homelessness among racial/ethnic minorities may bias residents against homeless persons, potentially reducing support for supportive housing policies[a]; municipal population demographics estimates are a proxy for demographics of the municipal homeless population[b]	Municipal statistical area (MSA) gross domestic product (Bureau of Economic Analysis 2017)	Municipal wealth is associated with greater provision of social services (De Benedictis-Kessner and Warshaw 2015; Peterson 1981)
Medicaid expansion (National Conference of State Legislatures 2018)	Medicaid expansion improved access to healthcare services for single adults and can also be used to pay for supportive housing services[c]	Percentage Latino (U.S. Census Bureau 2017)		MSA population (U.S. Census Bureau 2017)	Population may be related to rates of participation in supportive housing policy debates and stakeholder mobilization for/against supportive housing policies
State Level Supportive Housing Policy[d]	Additional state level policies targeting chronic homelessness may incentivize municipal supportive housing policy development	Percentage white (U.S. Census Bureau 2017)		Total chronically homeless (U.S. Department of Housing and Urban Development 2017c)	Numbers of chronically homeless persons by municipality; higher numbers of visibly homeless persons may incite cities to be more responsive to homelessness

(continued)

Table 3.1 CONTINUED

Political Institutions	Description	Social Construction	Description	Controls	Description
City Policy Conservatism (Warshaw and Tausanovitch 2015)	City-level ideal-point measure of public's conservatism; ideology is a strong factor of social policy, increased conservatism associated with lower social service provision (Grossman and Hopkins 2016)	Former Confederacy (Editors of Encyclopaedia Britannica 2019)	Given the policy histories of racial/ethnic marginalization, exploitation and criminalization[a] of racial/ethnic minority group members and Black Americans in particular in former confederate and southern states, it is reasonable to assume that these histories may play a role in shaping policies addressing chronic homelessness given the higher risk of homelessness faced by racial/ethnic minority group members	Total year-round permanent supportive housing beds (U.S. Department of Housing and Urban Development 2017c)	The total number of supportive housing beds by MSA[f]
Number of nonprofit health organizations (National Center for Charitable Statistics 2018)[g]	Proxy measure of the local Continuum of Care; measure of the average number of nonprofit healthcare providers per 10,000 people by MSA; decentralization influences policymaking processes	Southern City (U.S. Department of Commerce Economics and Statistics Administration 2010)		Total unsheltered chronically homeless (U.S. Department of Housing and Urban Development 2017c)	Numbers of chronically homeless persons who are unsheltered, by municipality; higher numbers of visibly homeless persons may incite cities to be more responsive to homelessness

Variable (source)	Description
Nonprofit health organization revenue (National Center for Charitable Statistics 2018)	Nongovernmental actor financing may influence policy outcomes; measure of nonprofit organizations per capita revenue by MSA
Religiosity (Association of Religion Data Archives 2010)	Religiosity intersects with ideology, notions of race/ethnicity, and deservedness (Weir and Schirmer 2018); measured by the rate of the churchgoing population, religiosity may indicate support toward, or away from municipal supportive housing policy, based on how it is associated with conservative ideology or animus towards outgroup members, or not
Continuum of Care (CoC) type (municipal arrangement)	Whether the Continuum of Care is organized within a major metropolitan area, or a small metropolitan area. Larger municipalities may have bigger budgets allowing them to spend more on social services.
Percentage of prisoners in private prisons (U.S. Department of Justice. Office of Justice Programs 2011)	Interest groups are able to influence political decision-making (Strach 2015). The relationship between chronic homelessness and incarceration may incentivize the private carceral state to retain and reincarcerate inmates; prison data were used in lieu of recent data on private jails, which is not available
Sanctuary City Status (U.S. Immigrations and Customs Enforcement 2017c)	Sanctuary city status is an indicator of social construction toward ethnic minority group members.[h]
State or regional Continuum of Care	The presence of a statewide or regional Continuum of Care responsible for a larger geographic area of the state that may coordinate with the local Continuum of Care and possibly improve policy capacity

(continued)

Table 3.1 CONTINUED

Political Institutions	Description	Social Construction	Description	Controls	Description
Tourism	Interest groups are able to influence political decision-making; tourism may be related to economic elite interests promoting reactionary policing as opposed to long-term housing investments (Nacgourney 2016)			State-level Dummy Variable	A state level dummy variable was included to control for differences across the states and to account for omitted variables.
				Winter temperature (National Centers for Environmental Information and National Oceanographic and Atmospheric Administration 2017)	The places with the highest rates of homelessness are concentrated along the coasts, many in warmer latitudes; control for geographic variation in rates of homelessness

[a]However, demographic information about this population is difficult to access. The U.S. Department of Housing and Urban Development collects demographic data during Point-in-Time homeless counts conducted by the Continuums of Care (Bishop et al. 2017). This includes racial and ethnic data, as reported in the Annual Homeless Assessment Report to Congress. As of 2019, however, racial and ethnic demographic data were not available in the publicly available HUD Point-in-Time data sets, although other demographic information is publicized such as age categories.
[b]However, using municipal demographic statistics may actually underestimate the effects of race on city policy choices, as ethnic minorities face greater risks of homelessness than whites as a product of historic wealth distributions and racial resentment (Bishop et al. 2017; Henwood et al. 2013).
[c]Medicaid itself cannot pay for housing or rent.

[d] See Appendix A for complete description of search strategy.

[e] Criminalization of minority group members may also be related to supportive housing policy decision-making. As discussed in Chapters 1 and 2, there is a long policy history of the criminalization of homelessness, which continues today, in part due to the social construction of persons experiencing chronic homelessness. While municipalities are incentivized to pursue supportive housing through federal regulation, they are also incentivized to move away from the default of criminalization. Therefore, cities with stronger histories of criminalization of out-group members may opt away from supportive housing in favor of the status quo of criminalization, as a product of path dependence and social construction of out-group members.

[f] Total number of supportive housing beds, a proxy measure for supportive housing implementation, may or may not be associated with supportive housing policy presence because of the many barriers that exist in allocating space for supportive housing or building new construction beyond municipal support.

[g] Because of the history of decentralization in homeless policy, measures of the level of nongovernmental activity (or here the Continuum of Care) is a critical component to understanding factors associated with homeless policy outcomes. A greater number of nongovernmental actors in the policy space may reflect lower governmental involvement in homeless policy or greater decentralization.

[h] For instance, sanctuary city status may be protective to minority group members, signaling more support for policies that protect racial/ethnic minority group members. Although sanctuary city status refers specifically to immigration status, the high rate of homelessness among minority groups and the overlap in social service needs among persons experiencing homelessness and other low-income groups may increase policy support for supportive housing in a case of support for a tangential policy, such as sanctuary city status, which is measured as a binary indicator (i.e., yes/no) for 2017 sanctuary city status.

may shape what policies actors pursue and therefore promote or dissuade preferences toward supportive housing policy. These include population measures of race/ethnicity, former confederacy, sanctuary city status, and religiosity. Control variables pertain to infrastructure, existing resources and need and include measures of the homeless population, municipal financial indicators, weather, and a dummy variable included for state effects.

Operationalization

This study applies two approaches to estimate political predictors of municipal supportive housing policy. The first is a set-theoretic approach using fsQCA (Ragin, Drass, and Davey 2006), beginning with a larger set of variables to deduce the *types* of municipalities, or characteristics of different types of municipalities, that are *most commonly* associated with supportive housing policy. FsQCA measures the proportions of the common types of characteristics in municipalities, stratified across the data set. If certain types of municipalities, or combinations of characteristics, are more predictive of municipal supportive housing policy, how common is this kind of city within the sample? For example, are some groupings of municipal characteristics associated with supportive housing very uncommon? Or are some groupings of characteristics associated with supportive housing more common? This gives us an idea of the overall heterogeneity or homogeneity between "types" or "exemplars" of municipalities within an outcome sample. Understanding this heterogeneity allows for more nuanced understanding of the different relationships between factors associated with a certain outcome. For example, some groupings of variables or municipal exemplars may represent a higher proportion of the sample than other combinations.

FsQCA also estimates the strength of the association between types of municipalities and the outcome of interest (Ragin 2014). Measuring the strength of the association is important because it allows us to identify municipal exemplars that are *very* predictive of supportive housing policy (rather than less predictive) and to understand how common these types of municipalities actually are. Overall, fsQCA adds value by looking at how different variables are associated in a particular type of municipal case rather than measuring average effects across all municipal cases in the data set. Focusing on mean effects alone may obscure this heterogeneity and therefore ignore important mechanisms or characteristics influencing an outcome. Identifying this variation is important, because it demonstrates that local governments may arrive at the same outcome as a result of different factors and processes. It is important to identify major trends that may apply to the majority of cases, through the use of average effects. Yet, it is equally as important to identify heterogeneity that may help us more completely understand the different processes involved in designing and delivering successful municipal approaches to chronic homelessness.

After fsQCA was used to identify the most common combinations of variables associated with each outcome, the most representative and most predictive groupings from each outcome set were applied in regression analysis to further test the relationships. With a binary outcome variable, logistic regression was used to understand the association of key individual variables with the outcome of municipal supportive housing policy (Hosmer and Lemeshow 2004). Logistic regression analysis is useful in this context because, as previously discussed, instead of highlighting heterogeneity within the sample, logistic regression analyzes mean associations of variables across the sample with the outcome of interest, allowing researchers to obtain a broad view of the factors associated with an outcome of interest. A broad analysis is an important first step in this novel research to identify factors associated with municipal supportive housing policy.[3] Using logistic regression in tandem with fsQCA provides both a broad and narrow view of the factors associated with an outcome of interest. Thus, comparing the results of the two approaches enhances the validity and reliability of the findings.

COMPARATIVE CASE STUDY DESIGN

As previously discussed, the fsQCA software (Ragin, Drass, and Davey 2006) traced the combinations of conditions associated with municipal homeless policy outcomes in the larger *n* sample—the presence or absence of a municipal-level supportive housing policy. This first step informs more precise case selection by maximizing variation across cases based on the groupings of variables associated with each case from the quantitative analysis, to identify the "diversity of factors" stratified across cases within an outcome of interest (Ragin 2014; Ragin, Drass, and Davey 2006). From there, I was able to control for a wider range of characteristics compared to typical case selection methodologies (Plümper, Troeger, and Neumayer 2019). I was also able to select on both independent variables of interest and the outcomes based on sample heterogeneity.

The comparative case study methodology is an ideal approach for understanding policy decision-making because it is imbued with inherent flexibility to use all relevant data and present it in a variety of ways. Not only can I select cases that are representative of the existing heterogeneity from the national sample to improve generalizability, but I can also conduct in-depth analyses of the processes at work in each city case. The qualitative analyses contextualize the findings from the quantitative work, especially in the absence of longitudinal data. The in-depth case studies enhance the quantitative analyses by providing a more nuanced understanding of the processes at work and their temporality, shaping municipal choices to engage in homeless policy governance, if at all, and subsequently why municipalities may or may not approach chronic homelessness through the evidence-based approach of supportive housing.

Case Selection

FsQCA software identified municipalities that were most representative of the common groupings of variables across the outcomes of interest, or "exemplars" of different types of municipalities—those that represent the highest proportion of the sample that are also the most predictive of the outcome—to facilitate municipal case selection.[4] The most representative cases can then be further stratified by independent variables of interest to control for factors across municipalities within the outcome set but also select upon independent variables of interest. I selected one case for municipalities *without* a municipal supportive housing policy, as there was less heterogeneity in this outcome set. This will be discussed in more detail later in the chapter. Two cases of municipalities with a supportive housing policy were selected to examine the effects of this heterogeneity on policy decision-making and implementation in municipalities with the same outcome.

As shown in Table 3.2, Shreveport, LA, was most representative of municipalities without a municipal level homeless policy, but with Medicaid expansion (representing 30% of cases *without* a municipal homeless policy). San Francisco, CA, was most representative of municipalities in the sample *with* a municipal homeless policy and with Medicaid expansion (representing 25% of cases with a municipal homeless policy). Atlanta, GA, acts as the control case to examine the variation in service access and policy conflict in a large municipality with a municipal homeless policy, in a state without Medicaid expansion (representing just over 25% of cases with a municipal homeless policy but without Medicaid expansion).

Table 3.2 CASE CHARACTERISTICS

Case	Municipal Level Supportive Housing Policy	Municipal Ideology	Municipality Size	Population Demographics	Municipal Fragmentation	Non-profit Health Organization Concentration	Winter Temperature	Rates of Chronic Homelessness	Medicaid expansion
Shreveport, LA	No	Conservative	Medium	Majority Black	Low	Low	High	Low	Yes
San Francisco, CA	Yes	Not conservative	Large	Minority Black	Low	Low	High	High	Yes
Atlanta, GA	Yes	Not conservative	Large	Majority Black	Medium	Low	High	High	No

Atlanta is categorized as having low municipal fragmentation in fuzzy set qualitative comparative analysis (fsQCA), as a result of having a comparatively low number of municipal governments within Fulton County, the county in which Atlanta primarily resides. I am classifying Atlanta in the case selection as having "medium" fragmentation as a result of the multiple, overlapping counties and subsequent municipal governments that make up the metropolitan statistical area of Atlanta, but are not counted in the census definition of municipal fragmentation. The fsQCA cut-off for high/low in the stratified, proportional sampling procedure is 0.5. See Appendix A for complete details about the variable coding for fsQCA and Appendix B for the details of the analysis.

Cases Without Municipal Level Supportive Housing Policy

Three municipalities were consistently representative of the major city types in the proportion of the sample absent supportive housing. These cases are Kalamazoo, MI; Shreveport, LA; and Provo, UT. Provo was present in fewer models, but the models it was present in were highly predictive and representative. However, Provo is a highly homogenous, religious[5] community, which may make Provo more of an outlying case. Kalamazoo may similarly face unobserved heterogeneity, as Kalamazoo was consistently representative in models of municipalities with low winter temperature. Municipalities with low winter temperature may inherently respond to homelessness in inherently different ways. Therefore, Kalamazoo may be less comparable to cases without cold winters. To improve comparability to the findings for municipalities *with* supportive housing policy, Shreveport was selected as the representative case for cities *without* municipal level supportive housing policy. Shreveport was also the municipal exemplar that was identified most often across all of the highly predictive and representative models.

Cases With Municipal Supportive Housing Policy

There were many cases consistently representative of the most common municipal types, within the outcome set of municipalities that have a supportive housing policy. Yet, of all of the cases listed, San Francisco occurred in most representative variations (see Appendix B for complete details on the stratified, proportional sampling analysis). Since San Francisco has a consistently high representation for nearly every variation of the common groupings of variables, I selected San Francisco as the most representative case for municipalities with a local level supportive housing policy.

Due to higher rates of heterogeneity in cases with municipal supportive housing policy, I am also selecting a second case. Atlanta has the same characteristics as San Francisco, controlling for all independent variables except three—Medicaid expansion, municipal fragmentation, and percentage of the population identifying as Black (see Table 3.2). This enhances my ability to select on independent variables of interest and compare the effects of this stratification between cases on municipal supportive housing policy development.

Qualitative Analytic Strategy for Comparative Case Studies

Qualitative case studies are a useful approach to enhance understanding of policy decision-making processes because they provide inherent flexibility to use all relevant data and present it in a variety of ways (Anckar 2008). Applying rigorously selected cases and in-depth qualitative analyses enhance quantitative findings by further examining the complex relationships and temporality of multiple factors affecting policy decision-making (Anckar 2008). In each case, I collected two types of qualitative data: interviews and textual document data. Interviews and document analysis add contextual grounding of the complicated relationships between the multiple factors at work and help tease apart political decision-making processes leading to the outcome with a greater level of detail (Collier 2011).

Interviews

A stratified sample of political actors involved in the policy decision-making process were recruited in each case. I conducted a total of 49 in-depth interviews across the three cases. Appendix C lists interviewees by case. Interviewee recruitment focused on the municipal level, although some state level bureaucrats involved in local-level initiatives were also interviewed. To determine appropriate categories of interviewees, municipal policy documents were used to outline the decision makers involved in local homeless and supportive housing policy. Five main categories of interviewees emerged from this outline: municipal bureaucrats, community-based organizations (which includes formal Continuum of Care governing organizations when the Continuum of Care is fully decentralized), elected municipal officials, law enforcement/public safety (includes local police, jail, and courts), and healthcare providers.

Interviews were conducted until saturation was achieved to enhance reliability (Fusch and Ness 2015).[6] A stratified sampling approach with the goal of saturation is much more effective in improving reliability by generating consistency in emergent themes across each group of actors (Rubin and Rubin 2011). Interviews were conducted in a semistructured format to allow for the exploration of ideas and a more genuine dialogue with interviewees, while utilizing a set of predetermined themes based on the research questions and factors of interest (Frechtling 2002; Rubin and Rubin 2011; see Appendixes D and E for the consent protocol and interview guide, respectively). Political actors were queried with a series of open-ended questions to engage them in sharing their experiences and perspectives on the policy decision-making process, including challenges and strategies employed or encountered in the context of the city's approach to chronic homelessness. To improve validity, the interviews were triangulated with official data from policy documents, such as floor debate transcripts or city council meeting transcripts.

Text Data

I collected archival documents from multiple sources at the state, local, and federal level to provide institutional and social context and intent behind decision-making. The body of text includes work at the state level on relevant policies such as Medicaid expansion and behavioral health services. The body of text included over 200 primary policy documents, with at least 50 policy documents per case. At the federal level, I used the publicly available from HUD (2019b and c) to collect Annual Action Plans from the Continuums of Care in each municipal case. The majority of texts are local-level documents related to local homeless policy decision-making, with a focus on addressing chronic homelessness as this is the topic of this research. Such documents include mayoral briefs or news releases; city council meeting minutes; notices of public comment; municipal supportive housing policies and accompanying local regulatory briefs, research, and reports; and any available documents from local law enforcement related to homelessness and chronic homelessness. In each city case, the documents collected range over many years to trace the policy histories and debates in each case effectively to understand the factors affecting formal municipal involvement in homeless policy and the decision to establish a municipal-level supportive housing policy.

Analytic Approach

I employed process tracing as the primary analytic approach. Process tracing is a systematic review of evidence across time, allowing for an analysis of the sequence of events and retrieval of key contextual information to divulge a causal mechanism (Bennett 2010; Collier 2011). The goal of process tracing is to document whether or not the sequence of events within the case fits those predicted by alternative explanations (Bennett 2010). The historical explanation allows for a deep understanding of the mechanism involved in the individual case, which helps develop larger theories about macrophenomena (Bennett 2009).

The document coding and interview coding occurred in an iterative process. An initial coding protocol in Appendix F was developed based on the literature. I conducted open coding to allow for other, non-predetermined themes to arise from the data. The coding protocol was then updated iteratively in response to themes derived from the process tracing analytic approach. Myself and a second coder—both PhD-trained political scientists—were used for consensus, enhancing measurement validity and establishing interrater reliability. Dedoose™ software was used to organize, code, map decision-making processes, and establish intercoder consensus for all interviews. I then triangulated between the archival documents with the interviews to effectively establish the sequence of events and actors involved in political decision-making and to validate the mechanisms and themes associated with the outcomes of interest (see Appendix G for details).

Cross-Case Analysis

By teasing out the complex processes involved in policy development, process tracing also helps examine the main factors at work and extract themes to compare the findings across individual cases. Comparing results across variant cases allows researchers to understand and theorize how political decision-making is influenced by contextual arrangements in each case—such as institutional structures, ideological, economic and social factors, and existing lateral policies—to better explain and theorize about the relationship between context and divergent policy outcomes (Mahoney and Thelen 2015). Pairing process tracing with the quantitative approach evaluating the national scope of municipal involvement in supportive housing policy lets us gain a deeper understanding of the mechanisms at work across outcomes and case type to better understand homeless policy outcomes and the developments leading up to related decisions.

CHAPTER 4

Measuring Municipal Participation in Homeless Governance

A National Perspective

When we attempt to understand why municipalities respond to chronic homelessness in different ways and why municipalities may leverage evidence-based strategies or not, we first need to know what is going on in municipalities around the United States. This chapter examines the national variation in municipal responses to chronic homelessness. Specifically, the goals of this chapter are (1) to identify the prevalence of municipal-level supportive housing policies among municipalities affected by homelessness in the United States and (2) to identify and examine the political factors associated with the presence of a municipal-level supportive housing policy.

These goals are critical for a number of reasons. First, most research on chronic homelessness focuses on identifying strategies that most effectively reduce chronic homelessness and improve health outcomes. This is very important research. However, to date, there has been almost no research on the political predictors (or other social or economic predictors) of the *adoption* of these evidence-based policies. Research has shown that the number of supportive housing units is not correlated with homelessness prevalence (T. Byrne et al. 2014). This would suggest that other factors, such as political predictors of policy adoption and implementation, might be affecting supportive housing development. This research intends to fill that gap. This is the first research to document municipal supportive

Ungoverned and Out of Sight. Charley E. Willison, Oxford University Press (2021). © Oxford University Press.
DOI: 10.1093/oso/9780197548325.003.0004

housing policy and evaluate the association between political and social factors and supportive housing policy in municipalities. Since these data have never before been collected, there are only cross-sectional data to draw from, and this research is therefore unable to evaluate temporality. However, identifying the factors associated with supportive housing policy presence in municipalities is a critical first step in ultimately understanding why supportive housing policies may or may not get implemented, as well as the types of places that may be more or less likely to adopt supportive housing policy approaches.

Second, the existence of a municipal level supportive housing policy presents evidence of coordination between the Continuum of Care and the municipal governments in supportive housing policy processes/efforts. The Continuum of Care, the national system for preventing and addressing homelessness, is a network of mainly nongovernmental community organizations, arranged at the municipal level that distribute funding and oversee local and regional homeless policy programming and service distribution (Jarpe, Mosley, and Smith 2019). Previous research has shown that most Continuums of Care tend not to coordinate with municipal-level governments (Jarpe, Mosley, and Smith 2019; Valero and Jang 2016), creating gaps in service delivery and implementation challenges. In response, the U.S. Department of Housing and Urban Development incentivizes coordination across the Continuums of Care and municipal governments, arguing that to deliver effective programming, there needs to be buy-in across these two sectors (U.S. Department of Housing and Urban Development Office of Policy Development and Research 2018). From a public health perspective, the presence of municipal-level supportive housing policies is also an indication of evidence-based policy adoption to address chronic homelessness effectively in urban areas.

The results show that most municipalities facing homelessness challenges do not have supportive housing policies. Of the municipalities in the data set, 40% had a municipal-level supportive housing policy. Three key factors are associated with municipal supportive housing policy: ideology; measures of the Continuum of Care including decentralization and capacity; and state politics. This research tells us that municipalities with a supportive housing policy are more likely to be liberal, sanctuary cities with less decentralized homeless programming and are located in states without Medicaid expansion.

Overall, the national data present a picture of a decentralized and fragmented policy space where local governments and the Continuums of Care are less likely to formally work together on evidence-based approaches to address chronic homelessness, thereby devolving solutions to chronic homelessness on the nongovernmental Continuums of Care. Additionally, these findings suggest that state policies may be less related to, and therefore possibly important for, municipal supportive housing policy efforts. The case studies in the next chapters going forward will tease out the implications of these findings to explore the mechanisms by which these policy interests are separate and the implications of decentralization and fragmentation for municipal supportive housing policy success.

DATA AND METHODS

A novel data set of 232 municipalities, representing two thirds of municipal Continuums of Care across the United States, was developed to document and measure municipal homeless policy choices and political factors associated with these choices. Municipal policies were selected from the municipal codes and regulations database Municode and cross-validated against city and county websites for each municipal Continuum of Care. Set theory and logistic regression were used to identify key variables associated with different policy outcomes and the heterogeneity and homogeneity between municipalities within the same outcome set based on the presence or absence of a local supportive housing policy (Hosmer and Lemeshow 2004; Ragin 2014). See Chapter 3 of this volume for complete methodology and detailed description of the data set and sample selection strategy.

Interrogating the distribution of municipal supportive housing policy gives us an indication of the scope of municipal investment in policies addressing chronic homelessness across the nation and begins to paint a picture of the similarities and differences between municipalities that are engaged in homelessness governance through evidence-based policy and how that engagement may align with other political factors including measures of intergovernmental relations and social construction.

DESCRIPTIVE RESULTS

This first section gives us an important overview of municipal participation in supportive housing policy or formal supportive housing policy responses to chronic homelessness by local governments. Shown in Table 4.1, 94 municipalities within the sample, or just over 40%, had a supportive housing policy in 2017. This finding indicates that the responsibility for homeless programming may fall primarily on the Continuum of Care or nongovernmental actors. This finding aligns with previous

Table 4.1 DESCRIPTIVE RESULTS—MUNICIPAL SUPPORTIVE HOUSING POLICIES

N Cases	Dependent Variable	Description
94	Supportive housing policy	Supportive housing addresses chronic homelessness by treating socioeconomic *and* physiological causes of homelessness by simultaneously providing housing and medical services; includes Housing First, but not exclusively.
138	No supportive housing policy	Municipalities found not to have some form of a supportive housing policy
232	Total	All municipalities in the sample

research, showing that 38% of Continuums of Care in 2014 were overseen by municipal actors, with government agencies accounting for just 17% of Continuums of Care membership overall (Jarpe, Mosley, and Smith 2019).

The results from the set theoretic analysis are shown in Figures 4.1 to 4.4. The set theoretic approach sorts through combinations of the selected variables to show us results revealing the different types of municipalities *within* the outcome set (presence or absence of municipal supportive housing policy) that both occur most frequently in the outcome set *and* accurately predict the outcome. Figures 4.1 to 4.4 report the top outcomes (most common and most predictive) that were deduced from the minimization procedure (described in detail in Chapter 3). Parsimonious solutions are also included. Parsimonious solutions are further minimizations within municipal types that may be more predictive than the larger combination of characteristics, as a result of the inherent trade-offs between proportion of the sample represented, predictiveness, and the number of parameters included in each model.

There are a few important findings from this analysis. First, as shown in Figure 4.1, for understanding municipalities with supportive housing policy, the types of municipalities that are *most common* and *most predictive* of supportive housing policy represent at least one fourth of the municipalities with a municipal supportive housing policy. This tells us that there is a lot of variation in the characteristics across the majority of municipalities with a local supportive housing policy but that 25% share similar characteristics. By comparison, among municipalities *without* a supportive housing policy, the greatest proportion of municipalities with similar characteristics predictive of the outcome set is over 50% of the

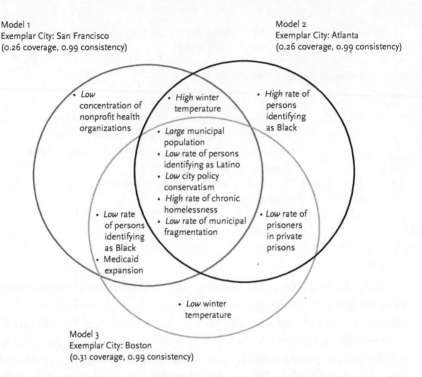

Model 1
Exemplar City: San Francisco
(0.26 coverage, 0.99 consistency)

Model 2
Exemplar City: Atlanta
(0.26 coverage, 0.99 consistency)

- *Low* concentration of nonprofit health organizations
- *High* winter temperature
- *High* rate of persons identifying as Black
- *Large* municipal population
- *Low* rate of persons identifying as Latino
- *Low* city policy conservatism
- *High* rate of chronic homelessness
- *Low* rate of municipal fragmentation
- *Low* rate of persons identifying as Black
- Medicaid expansion
- *Low* rate of prisoners in private prisons
- *Low* winter temperature

Model 3
Exemplar City: Boston
(0.31 coverage, 0.99 consistency)

Figure 4.1 Characteristics of municipalities with municipal supportive housing policy. Coverage refers to the proportion of the sample represented by the exemplar 0–1 or the representativeness of the case. Consistency refers to the predictability of the exemplar for the outcome set, 0–1. See Appendix B for complete details on the set-theoretic approach. *Source:* Willison (2020).

outcome set (across all of the most common and most predictive models; see Figure 4.5). This disparity suggests that there are more differences between municipalities that have supportive housing policies and comparably more similarities between municipalities that don't have a local supportive housing policy. Alternatively, this may indicate that the analysis could be strengthened by including additional variables to try to account for currently unobserved heterogeneity among municipalities with a local supportive housing policy.[1]

Overall, the set theory results tell an important story about the types of municipalities that employ supportive housing policy compared to those that do not. Municipalities with a supportive housing policy are more likely to be in states with Medicaid expansion; have high rates of chronic homelessness; a large municipal population; lower rates of nonprofit health organizations; and higher mean winter temperatures. These municipalities are more likely to have lower populations of Black and Latino residents, lower city conservatism, less municipal governmental fragmentation,

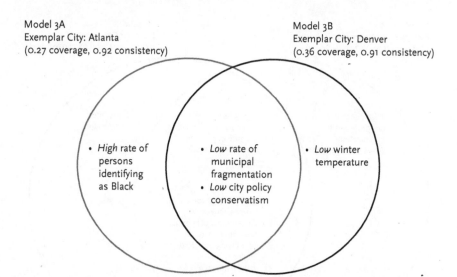

Model 3A
Exemplar City: Atlanta
(0.27 coverage, 0.92 consistency)

Model 3B
Exemplar City: Denver
(0.36 coverage, 0.91 consistency)

- *High* rate of persons identifying as Black

- *Low* rate of municipal fragmentation
- *Low* city policy conservatism

- *Low* winter temperature

Figure 4.2 Characteristics of municipalities with municipal supportive housing policy—parsimonious models. Coverage refers to the proportion of the sample represented by the exemplar 0–1 or the representativeness of the case. Consistency refers to the predictability of the exemplar for the outcome set, 0–1. See Appendix B for complete details on the set-theoretic approach.
Source: Willison (2020).

and lower rates of nonprofit healthcare organizations. For municipalities *without* supportive housing policies, the majority are places with high rates of municipal governmental fragmentation, higher city conservatism, and large population sizes. Most municipalities without supportive housing have fewer chronically homeless persons and, like municipalities with supportive housing, also have lower rates of ethnic minorities and fewer non-profit health organizations.

Municipalities With Supportive Housing Policies

Based on these results, the most consistent municipal exemplars with the highest proportion of the sample represented and predictive of outcome set also do not present an unexpected picture. Regarding institutional resources, Medicaid expansion was predictive of supportive housing policy presence across most city types. States may make more resources available if there is a high number of municipalities in need and policy preferences align. As a counterfactual, municipalities may be more likely to engage in supportive housing policy if they believe they can leverage state resources.

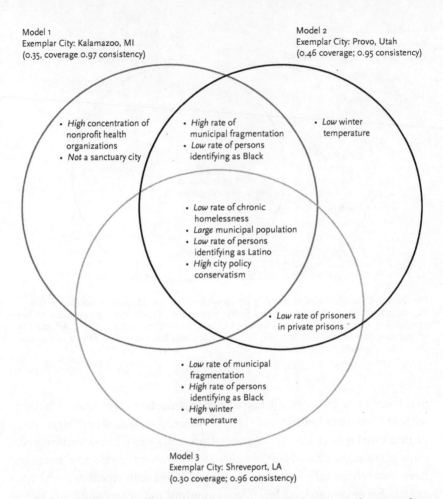

Model 1
Exemplar City: Kalamazoo, MI
(0.35, coverage 0.97 consistency)

Model 2
Exemplar City: Provo, Utah
(0.46 coverage; 0.95 consistency)

- *High* concentration of nonprofit health organizations
- *Not* a sanctuary city

- *High* rate of municipal fragmentation
- *Low* rate of persons identifying as Black

- *Low* winter temperature

- *Low* rate of chronic homelessness
- *Large* municipal population
- *Low* rate of persons identifying as Latino
- *High* city policy conservatism

- *Low* rate of prisoners in private prisons

- *Low* rate of municipal fragmentation
- *High* rate of persons identifying as Black
- *High* winter temperature

Model 3
Exemplar City: Shreveport, LA
(0.30 coverage; 0.96 consistency)

Figure 4.3 Characteristics of municipalities without municipal supportive housing policy. Coverage refers to the proportion of the sample represented by the exemplar 0–1 or the representativeness of the case. Consistency refers to the predictability of the exemplar for the outcome set, 0–1. See Appendix B for complete details on the set-theoretic approach. *Source*: Willison (2020).

The low concentration of nonprofit health organizations shown in Figure 4.1 (Model 1), as a measure of decentralization, aligns theoretically. If municipalities are engaged in supportive housing policy, this may translate into greater centralization, namely, coordination of services through municipal government compared to nongovernmental community actors. Therefore, we may see lower rates of nonprofit health organizations overall in municipalities with these policies. We may also potentially see lower nonprofit revenue as an effect of greater centralization in municipalities with supportive housing policy.

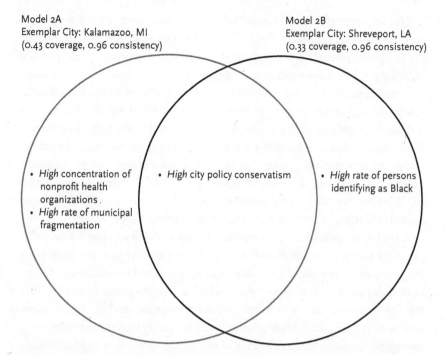

Model 2A
Exemplar City: Kalamazoo, MI
(0.43 coverage, 0.96 consistency)

Model 2B
Exemplar City: Shreveport, LA
(0.33 coverage, 0.96 consistency)

- *High* concentration of nonprofit health organizations.
- *High* rate of municipal fragmentation

- *High* city policy conservatism

- *High* rate of persons identifying as Black

Figure 4.4 Characteristics of municipalities without municipal supportive housing policy—parsimonious models. Coverage refers to the proportion of the sample represented by the exemplar 0–1 or the representativeness of the case. Consistency refers to the predictability of the exemplar for the outcome set, 0–1. See Appendix B for complete details on the set-theoretic approach.
Source: Willison (2020).

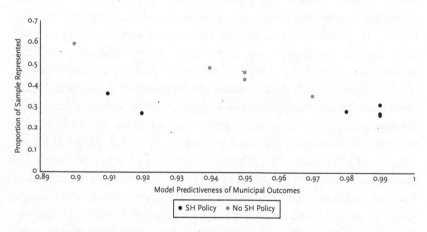

Figure 4.5 Generalizability and predictiveness of municipal supportive housing policy exemplar models.

Not surprisingly, liberal municipalities are more predictive of municipal supportive housing policy. Regarding institutional structures, lower municipal government fragmentation is commonly predictive of supportive housing policies. Lower municipal fragmentation may work in similar ways as municipalities *without* supportive housing, where more streamlined governmental structures might make policy adoption easier. This may be indicative of greater ability to coordinate between Continuum of Cares and local government to establish a municipal-level supportive housing policy. Lower fragmentation appears to be predictive conditional on low city policy conservatism, as shown in Figure 4.2 (Model 3, Parsimonious A and B). This also aligns with traditional ideological notions of centralization or decentralization of welfare state activities (Pierson 1995).

A higher percentage of persons identifying as Black and low winter temperature also seem to work (separately) in conjunction with low municipal fragmentation and low city policy conservatism to be predictive of supportive housing policy (Figure 4.2, Model 3, Parsimonious A and B). This may be a product of lower municipal fragmentation and liberal ideology across *most* cases, here highlighting heterogeneity across some cases with divergent characteristics of colder winter temperatures or municipalities with higher rates of minority group members that also adopt supportive housing policies (in municipalities that are both liberal and less fragmented).[2]

Municipalities Without Supportive Housing

Based on these results (see Figures 4.3 and 4.4), the most consistent municipal exemplars (groupings of municipal characteristics) with the highest proportion of the sample represented and predictive of outcome set do not present an unexpected picture. Regarding political institutions, municipalities without supportive housing are more likely to be municipalities with greater municipal fragmentation. Municipal fragmentation is particularly predictive of municipalities without a supportive housing policy in the presence of greater conservatism and a higher rate of nonprofit healthcare providers (shown in Figure 4.3, Model 1; Figure 4.4, Model 1 Parsimonious). A higher proportion of nonprofit healthcare providers and conservative ideology fits with conceptions of neoliberalism and the traditional mechanisms for providing homeless services, which were historically based on neoliberal principles and a devolution to nongovernmental actors. Thus, more conservative municipalities may be more likely to adhere to neoliberal principles, retaining high levels of nonprofit service delivery. Municipal fragmentation may interact with this, making any interest in moving toward a municipal supportive housing policy less likely due to decentralized policy promulgation processes.

Alternative models (.24, .96) of Figure 4.3 (Model 3) showed there may be an overall lack of investment in social services by conservative municipalities, possibly leading to an overall lower concentration of non-profit healthcare organizations among municipalities without supportive housing policy. Further, lower rates of chronic homelessness paired with conservative ideology may promote limited investment in social services when the salience of homelessness aligns with conservative ideals of welfare systems. An absence of existing networks of social service organizations may also have the inverse effect on the adoption of supportive housing policies, if the absence of such a network prevents coalition-building by groups that might have a greater interest in promoting supportive housing solutions.

Overall, some interesting factors emerge from the findings from the set theoretic analyses of municipal exemplars with and without supportive housing policy: measures of higher levels of delegated state activity and municipal fragmentation in municipalities without supportive housing policy compared to municipalities *with* supportive housing policy. While the absence of a municipal supportive housing policy acts as a proxy for *formal* municipal involvement in homeless policy governance, measures of larger nongovernmental Continuum of Care activity may also indicate less coordination between Continuums and municipal governments overall, even absent formal supportive housing policy.

LOGISTIC REGRESSION RESULTS—AVERAGE TRENDS

The results from the logistic regression appear in Table 4.2. This model measures the associations of the independent variables of interest with the outcome, the presence of a municipal supportive housing policy. The logistic regression model includes the control variables,[3] a state-level dummy variable to control for state-level effects, and the variables from the main city types in the set theoretic analysis that had the highest representation in the city types across the outcome set. The complete list of variables included in the final model are listed in Table 4.2.

For sensitivity analysis, the variables that fell out of the set theoretic analyses were also run individually along with the main logit model (state-level supportive housing policy, tourism, Continuum of Care types, etc.). These variables were not significant. Total permanent supportive housing

Table 4.2 LOGISTIC REGRESSION RESULTS ON SUPPORTIVE HOUSING POLICY PRESENCE

Independent Variable	Coefficient	Odds Ratio
Medicaid expansion	−1.093*	.335
Total municipal fragmentation	−0.009	
Number of nonprofit health organizations	−0.331*	.718
Nonprofit health organization revenue	0.007*	1.007
Percentage private prisoners	6.085	
City policy conservatism	−4.071***	.017
Winter temperature	0.982	
Gross domestic product	−0.001	
Population	−0.005	
Percentage Black	−0.017	
Percentage Latino	0.035*	1.035
Sanctuary city	2.189***	8.928
Total permanent supportive housing beds	−0.000	
Total chronically homeless	0.002	

Odds ratios only show for statistically significant results. *$P < 0.05$. **$P < 0.01$. ***$P < 0.001$. Pseudo-$R^2 \geq$ 0.3154.

beds was also included in the regression even though it was not predictive in the set theoretic analysis as an important alternative measure of supportive housing policy support.

The results of the logistic regression mostly align with the results from the set theory analysis in terms of the associations between intergovernmental relations and municipal policy outcomes. The measures of nonprofit activity as a measure of decentralization or the Continuum of Care align with the set theoretic results for supportive housing policy. The number of nonprofit health organizations within a municipality is negatively and significantly associated with municipal supportive housing policy. Municipalities with higher proportions of nonprofit health organizations are about 30% less likely to have a municipal supportive housing policy. Theoretically, this aligns with notions of coordination and neoliberalism; greater numbers of nonprofits may create coordination challenges, while greater nonprofit presence aligns with historic conservative effort to decentralize homeless policy, which may subvert local government efforts (Cronley 2010; Soss, Fording, and Schram 2011; Willison 2017). It is important to note that causality may be bidirectional. A greater number of

nonprofits could be indicative of conservative trends pushing more resources away from centralized municipal efforts. Alternatively, a greater
number of nonprofits may be a historic effect that subsequently creates
challenges to generating a municipal response.

The relationship between nonprofit revenue and supportive housing
offers different insights. Nonprofit health organization revenue is positively and statistically significantly associated with municipal supportive
housing policy although the relationship is small (municipalities with
higher nonprofit health revenue are about 1% more likely to have a municipal supportive housing policy). This result suggests greater community or
municipal support for nonprofits, which could be indicative of an overall
greater municipal role in homeless policy. This relationship too, however,
may also be bidirectional. Greater nonprofit revenue may signal a stronger
stakeholder response by nonprofits, generating support for municipal supportive housing, as opposed to governmental initiation.

The city-types analysis differs from the logit in state-level policy and in
the relationships with the control variables. Regarding state-level policy,
Medicaid expansion runs in the opposite direction than anticipated theoretically. Municipalities in states with Medicaid expansion are nearly 70%
less likely to have a municipal supportive housing policy. This result is not
entirely surprising. This finding may indicate greater heterogeneity among
municipalities adopting supportive housing policy; for example, this may
be capturing divergence between state and municipal politics where large
municipalities in conservative states that oppose Medicaid expansion may
trend more liberal and be more likely to adopt supportive housing policies
(Miami, FL; Austin, TX; Nashville, TN; Atlanta, GA; etc.). This finding may
obscure other heterogeneity related to Medicaid waivers. For example,
Medicaid waivers can fund different types of supportive services in supportive housing (Alderwick, Hood-Ronick, and Gottlieb 2019). Different
municipalities have utilized waivers to supplement municipal efforts (e.g.,
Whole Person Care in San Francisco). Further research evaluating the relationship between different types of state level Medicaid waivers and local
supportive housing policy may shed light on the mechanisms between
Medicaid funding and local supportive housing policy.

There are somewhat mixed results in relation to control variables, where
two results differ between the set theory analysis and the logit analysis.
Municipal population shows a slightly negative but statistically significant
association with supportive housing policy. This result may be affected by
slightly greater heterogeneity in size of municipalities adopting supportive
housing compared to municipalities that do not. The other result that differs
between the two analyses is the percentage of the population identifying as

Latino. Having a higher percentage of Latino residents is positively and statistically significantly associated with municipal supportive housing policy. Municipalities with a higher percentage of the population identifying as Latino are 4% more likely to have a supportive housing policy. This association may be accounting for unobserved heterogeneity. There may be a diffusion effect of supportive housing policies across southwestern states where there are a higher proportion of Latino residents. There may also be an effect here of homeless rates correlating with percentage Latino, since Latino residents face a greater risk of homelessness compared to white counterparts (Fusaro, Levy, and Shaefer 2018).

Finally, two variables are strongly and significantly associated with municipal supportive housing policy. Both of these results also align with the set theory results. More conservative municipalities are about 98% less likely to have a supportive housing policy. This result is not surprising. Causality here, too, most likely runs in both directions. Conservative ideology may foster less support for supportive housing policy. Alternatively, conservative preferences fostering institutional barriers to supportive housing—such as municipal fragmentation and decentralization—may make any reduced ideological opposition to supportive housing, specifically, insufficient to overcome entrenched historical challenges.

Second, sanctuary cities have a positive and significant association with municipal supportive housing policy. Sanctuary city status is employed as a proxy measure of the city's perspective of ethnic minority persons as deserving or undeserving of governmental resources and protections, which may factor into city policy preferences for chronically homeless persons, a disproportionate proportion of whom are racial/ethnic minorities (Bishop et al. 2017b; Fusaro, Levy, and Shaefer 2018). Thus, the predictive nature of sanctuary city status for supportive housing policy is not surprising. This is also not surprising given the trend in liberal cities adopting sanctuary city status (Mehrotra and Larson 2017; U.S. Immigration and Customs Enforcement 2017a,b) and the association between liberal ideology and supportive housing policy adoption.

What is surprising is that sanctuary city status is much more predictive of municipal level supportive housing policy than local ideology. Sanctuary cities are 8.9 times the odds as likely to have a municipal supportive housing policy. The stark difference in these findings suggests that there is something different, perhaps beyond ideology, that is related to sanctuary city status that may strongly promote municipal level supportive housing policy.

The relationship between sanctuary city status and supportive housing policy may be bidirectional and may be related to local safety nets. Both municipal level supportive housing policy and sanctuary city status require buy-in and resources, at least to some degree, from local government actors. Both policies may engender greater municipal involvement in local safety net resources. Therefore, any expansion or relative strength of the existing safety net as signaled by either policy may create opportunities for other social welfare policies relying on similar safety net services to emerge. Alternatively, sanctuary city status may be a more accurate measure of municipal ideology compared to the current measure, potentially capturing ideological heterogeneity not fully captured in the existing measure.

SUMMARY AND POLICY IMPLICATIONS

These results have important implications for homeless policy. The first is the ability to describe the policy landscape by understanding the degree to which local governments may be involved in supportive housing policy. This research finds that just 40% of local governments in the sample have a supportive housing policy. Jarpe, Mosley, and Smith (2019) showed that 38% of Continuums of Care had local government as the primary governing structure in 2014. While this may suggest a marginal increase in local governmental participation, this research indicates a low-level of formal involvement by municipal governments in supportive housing policy when compared to norms of governance for public health and behavioral healthcare. Going forward, more research should be conducted to examine the implications of limited municipal involvement in supportive housing policy and identify other measures of degrees of municipal participation in homeless policy.

Due to data limitations, this research is cross-sectional, which constrains the ability to leverage temporal research designs that would provide insight into *why* local governments choose to participate in supportive housing policy or not. Where this research adds substantial value is that this is the first research investigating the relationships between different political, social, and economic factors and the presence of municipal supportive housing policy. Identifying the factors associated with municipal supportive housing policy presence is a first step in explaining why supportive housing policies may or may not get implemented, as well as the types of places that may be more or less likely to adopt supportive housing policy approaches.

Four key factors are associated with municipal supportive housing policy: ideology, measures of decentralization, state politics, and social construction. This research tells us that municipalities with a supportive housing policy are more likely to be liberal, sanctuary cities with less decentralized homeless programming that are located in states without Medicaid expansion. This has important policy implications and raises important questions about the relative separation of municipal governmental responses to chronic homelessness compared to the decentralized history of homelessness policy and programming in the United States (Jones 2015; Lee and Mcguire 2017) as well as the role of social construction in policy processes regarding municipal approaches to chronic homelessness.

First, regarding decentralization and state politics, many foundations of health policy that are touted in other areas of health services research may be less applicable in approaches to chronic homelessness. This includes state-level activities such as Medicaid expansion and the role of local governments as the primary arbiters of public health promotion, programming, and governance. Therefore, policymakers urging state-level coordination to address municipal homelessness or advocating for Medicaid expansion resources as a game changer for supportive housing efforts should consider that municipalities may make policy choices based on other factors. Future research should examine why Medicaid may be less consequential for local supportive housing policy.

Second, the measures of social construction in both analyses indicate important relationships between municipal supportive housing policy and perceptions of persons at risk of chronic homelessness (which will be explored further in the following case study chapters). The negative association between municipal fragmentation—a measure of the number of municipal governments in a county area, most often used as a mechanism by elites to create segregated jurisdictions—and municipal supportive housing policy in the set theoretic analyses provides evidence for the presence of elite interests in supportive housing policy processes that may be related to municipal supportive housing outcomes. Although these relationships couldn't be fully tested here due to data limitations, the findings support the main argument that the lack of coordination or separation between policy interests—the state, Continuum of Care, municipal government, and local elites—is related to whether or not a municipality has a supportive housing policy. The case studies expand these findings from the national data, temporally, to explain the mechanisms involved in municipal supportive housing policy decision-making.

CHAPTER 5

The Integrated State

San Francisco and Challenges for Policy Implementation

WHAT'S HAPPENING IN SAN FRANCISCO?

This chapter focuses on San Francisco, a case with strong municipal involvement in supportive housing policy and homeless policy governance, where the local government is the institution responsible for designing and implementing homeless policy in San Francisco. This institutional structure allows San Francisco to coordinate with other relevant municipal offices to promote evidence-based, supportive housing policy efforts. This chapter first examines why San Francisco's homeless governance system became integrated into local government and why San Francisco adopted a municipal level supportive housing policy. The chapter then focuses on explaining the lingering policy conflicts between the city of San Francisco, local elites, and the state of California that build barriers to implementing supportive housing policy in San Francisco and mitigating the city's homelessness crisis.

Introducing San Francisco

San Francisco is the fourth largest city in California, located on the northwest coast (Cubit 2020). San Francisco has a population of 883,000 residents (Data USA 2020b). The poverty rate in San Francisco is 11.7%, just below the national average of 13% (Data USA 2020b). Always a leader

Ungoverned and Out of Sight. Charley E. Willison, Oxford University Press (2021). © Oxford University Press.
DOI: 10.1093/oso/9780197548325.003.0005

in healthcare sciences, San Francisco's economy over the last decade has increasingly shifted toward the tech industry, although healthcare remains the second largest employer (Data USA 2020b; McNeill 2016). The largest proportion of San Francisco's population identifies as white, 40%; Asian, 34.1%; Hispanic or Latino about 12%; with black residents making up less than 5% of the population respectively (Data USA 2020b). According to the U.S. Department of Housing and Urban Development (HUD), there were 6,775 persons experiencing homelessness in San Francisco in 2015 (HUD 2015e). In 2018, there were 6,857 (HUD 2018e).

San Francisco, CA, serves as the representative case for municipalities *with* a municipal government level supportive housing policy. Twenty-five percent of the cities in the national data set (see Chapter 3 of this volume) with a supportive housing policy matched the same criteria (variables) as San Francisco. San Francisco also serves as the comparison case to Atlanta, GA (see Chapter 6 of this volume). Both cities have a municipal level supportive housing policy and are comparable across many characteristics (see Chapter 3 of this volume for case comparison details) but differ in two important ways: Atlanta is majority Black whereas San Francisco is majority white, and Georgia has not expanded Medicaid while California has. San Francisco and Atlanta provide an understanding of the *different ways* similar cities may end up with similar or dissimilar policies and the important role of different political institutions and policy histories in homeless policy decision-making and implementation.

San Francisco exemplifies the importance of the role of stakeholder compositions, the political economy, and recognizing and addressing implementation problems in public health policy. San Francisco stands as a case where the unified city and county have made significant contributions to addressing chronic homelessness. San Francisco's Continuum of Care (CoC),[1] the governing structures designated by the federal government to design and implement homelessness policy, as mentioned is integrated into municipal government, and the city has had a Housing First policy since the mid-1990s (Department of Homelessness and Supportive Housing and City and County of San Francisco 2019). San Francisco has an impressive amount of policy capacity expertise, municipal fiscal resources, and intergovernmental support to address homelessness that should have positioned it at the forefront of the supportive housing movement in the United States.

And for a time, it was. Yet substantial changes to San Francisco's political economy paired with the policy histories of limited governmental involvement in homeless policy in the United States created the perfect storm of implementation problems. San Francisco relies primarily (San

Francisco Budget and Legislative Analyst's Office 2016, 17) on municipal funding for homelessness programming with limited state-level support and exists in a political economy where wealthy residents—businesses and homeowners—dominate decision-making and stagnate municipal programming efforts. As a result, San Francisco has now become known for its devastating, and public, homelessness crisis.

Today, San Francisco's homelessness rate and chronic homelessness rate are increasing.[2] The city faces serious shortages of any affordable housing let alone supportive housing (San Francisco Budget and Legislative Analyst's Office 2016). San Francisco is a case study in political participation and implementation. Even when the perfect set up exists, things may not go as planned. In San Francisco's case, continued independent, or uncoordinated, policy approaches, by the state, local government, and economic elites, have contributed to the deep implementation challenges by generating perpetual policy conflict between the preferences, mechanisms, and intended policy goals and outcomes of policies pursued by local government, the state, and economic elites. The case of San Francisco shows that reduced coordination between these competing interests and their policy approaches—engendering participatory equity in homeless policy processes, making such policies less responsive to target populations and inhibiting implementation as a result of policy conflict—reduces the policy opportunities for publicly funded, evidence-based efforts. San Francisco is a case that may increasingly apply to other major cities in the United States facing housing crises.

Multiple, Competing Approaches to Homelessness in San Francisco

As mentioned, San Francisco has integrated the Continuum of Care into municipal government. This is the same model as Atlanta and is the opposite of Shreveport. Here, the Continuum of Care is a part of San Francisco's municipal bureaucracy. This institutional arrangement has given the Continuum of Care greater participatory equity in municipal policy debates, the ability to coordinate Continuum of Care policy activities with other city policies and departments related to homelessness such as policing, and the ability for the Continuum of Care to lobby for and leverage municipal funding resources.

Despite this integration, the other two policy interests—the state and economic elites—remain separate and create tension for the municipal Continuum of Care initiatives as a result of directly conflicting or misaligned policy goals. The State of California is identified as separate because it designs and delivers policies affecting supportive housing initiatives through different processes and to different ends. The state-level policy mechanisms are organized primarily around state and federal actors for decision-making purposes, although implementation is beginning to involve more local actors (San Francisco Department of Public Health 2017). The state-level policy goals remain misaligned from local homeless and supportive housing policy goals as the state goals focus mostly on medical needs as opposed to pairing housing with medical needs. This leads to programming that does not work with or adequately address the reality of chronic homelessness. Future integration of the state and local policy decision-making and implementation through Medicaid Innovation Waivers[3] may help to align the policy mechanisms and goals (San Francisco Department of Public Health 2017).

As the next two case studies will detail (Chapters 6 and 7, this volume), in San Francisco, "organized elites" are notably different from organized, economic elites in Atlanta and Shreveport. In San Francisco, compared to Atlanta and Shreveport, elite interests appear to be comprised of wealthy individuals (i.e., independent citizens) as to opposed corporate interests. Urban politics literature demonstrates that homeowners, particularly white, wealthy homeowners, drive local segregation through restrictive zoning activities, which constrains housing supply and promotes housing policy implementation problems (Bates and Santerre 1994; Einstein, Glick, and Palmer 2019; Trounstine 2019, 2020). Where this description would typically seem to include "citizens" as the general public, and perhaps not a minority group of wealthy individuals with a concentrated amount of power, San Francisco, as an urban area, stands in contrast.

The definition of "elite" in social sciences is a widely used term to describe the rule of a minority over the majority of the population (Zannoni 1978). The second distinction of "elite" is the existence of criteria to separate the minority from the majority (Zannoni 1978). In San Francisco's case, this distinction is income. As will be discussed in the coming sections, the city and county of San Francisco is an increasingly, economically homogenous area concentrated with wealthy individuals. In the city of San Francisco moderate-income households (80%–120% area median income [AMI]) have declined at double the rate of the Bay Area (San Francisco Department of Planning 2018, 30). Simultaneously, since 2000, the population of San Francisco residents with income over 200% of the AMI has increased by nearly 250% (San Francisco Department of Planning 2018, 30). Forty-seven percent of San Francisco residents as of 2015 earn 120% of the AMI or more, with 30% earning over 200% AMI. Sixty percent of homeowners in the city of San Francisco are residents earning over 120%

AMI. In effect, wealthy individuals who comprise a minority of Americans, and a minority of earned incomes in San Francisco (Rahaim et al. 2018, 32), now comprise the majority of landowners in San Francisco. Therefore, the high concentration of economic power among San Francisco property owners distinguishes them as economic elites. This definition matters because of the subsequent amount of political power stemming from wealthy property owners in San Francisco.

Economic elites' interests directly conflict with local supportive housing policy efforts. Elites also exert tension on local policies to stray from their intended goals. Further, elites place pressure on the integration between municipal actors and the Continuum of Care. Elites move their influence through informal policy processes that direct elite preferences through police activity and elected officials. This policy process is very different from both the state and integrated local government/Continuum of Care policy processes. The goals elites seek are also very different. Elites seek to address undesirable behaviors and visibility associated with homelessness as opposed to designing evidence-based approaches to address the causes of homelessness and chronic homelessness or policies aligning with *negative* social construction of persons experiencing homelessness (see Chapter 2, this volume). This direct policy conflict between the structural interests creates a fracturing in the policy spaces, where the municipal Continuum of Care is attempting to coordinate long-term solutions to homelessness across city services, including policing, and elite preferences often stymy these solutions by demanding short-term solutions to behaviors associated with chronic homelessness and interfering with existing regulatory policy.

HOW DID SAN FRANCISCO GET A SUPPORTIVE HOUSING POLICY? SHIFTING INTERGOVERNMENTAL RELATIONS AND HISTORIC POLICY CAPACITY

Before examining ongoing tensions in San Francisco's approaches to chronic homelessness, we will examine why San Francisco has an integrated Continuum of Care and municipal level Housing First policy approach. Political mobilization or policy capacity for homelessness and supportive housing is necessary but may not be sufficient for adopting a municipal-level supportive housing policy. Institutional changes may also be required to shift perceived responsibility for a historically decentralized policy area, or incentivize municipal actors to participate in a policy space they have historically had no role in. In San Francisco, despite substantial growth in municipal investment in housing and supportive services during the HIV/AIDS crisis, the city did not establish a formal municipal role governing homelessness services until after the State of California mandated reorganization of behavioral health services to be governed by counties as opposed to community-based, nongovernmental actors (San Francisco Budget and Legislative Analyst's Office 2016, 4). San Francisco acts as an example of the important role political institutions play in shaping policy decision-making and policy change. It may not be enough to have motivated political actors, knowledgeable bureaucrats, and strong funding sources to implement a policy. If structural responsibility for certain policy programming exists outside of the role of government, or is designated to other actors, government may be less incentivized to play a direct role even in cases where policy salience is high, the problem stream is strong, and all other resources align (Kingdon 1990).

In San Francisco, archival and interview analyses identified two main factors influencing San Francisco's buy-in to participate in supportive housing and homelessness policy and formally align with the Continuum of Care: (1) political mobilization spurring policy capacity development during the HIV/AIDS crisis and (2) institutional restructuring when the State of California shifted the organizational responsibility for behavioral healthcare from local nongovernmental actors to counties. Overall, the relationship between the development of strong policy capacity paired with structural realignment led to the development of San Francisco's municipal Continuum of Care and municipal level supportive housing policy.

Political Mobilization and Policy Capacity

Nearly all interviewees, along with archival analyses and extant literature, documented strong policy capacity and political mobilization around issues related to homelessness in San Francisco in the early 1990s. Understanding the political mobilization related to homelessness in San Francisco in the 1980s through the early 1990s is important because it documents the progressive relationship between increasing salience of homelessness with simultaneous policy capacity development, or San Francisco's increasing role in homelessness responses. This research argues that San Francisco's policy capacity surrounding homelessness was a necessary condition for municipal policy adoption, and ultimately, the interaction between strong policy capacity and the institutional restructuring allowed for San Francisco to develop a municipal supportive housing policy. Without developing strong policy expertise, restructuring the responsibility for behavioral healthcare may not have been a strong enough incentive for San Francisco to develop a municipal response to homelessness.

Interviewees stated that San Francisco was one of the first cities to establish supportive housing as a priority in the 1990s. "So the city [San Francisco] was relatively early with Philly and NYC very early out of the gate to do harm reduction or HF [Housing First] model, jump started in late 1990s."[4] As a progressive city with a wealthy tax base and a homelessness problem, San Francisco was active in addressing homelessness and adopting evidence-based strategies to do so (McGarry 2008). San Francisco's engagement in homelessness was related to local ideology and local political capacity surrounding homelessness. The political capacity stemmed from a strong advocacy and service provider network that put the city in a clear position to address homelessness through a social services framework (Blair 2016). Many of these provider networks and advocacy groups related to healthcare stemmed from development and mobilization during the AIDS outbreak in the 1980s.

San Francisco was at the epicenter of the AIDS outbreak in the 1980s (H. Byrne 2018). San Francisco's small geographic footprint paired with the thriving gay community made the epidemic very salient in the community (H. Byrne 2018, Episode 3). As a liberal city that had been in the forefront of the civil rights movement, Vietnam protests, and gay rights movement, San Francisco was ideologically positioned to tackle the outbreak (Luce 2013). Politicians from the 1980s through the 1990s were heavily involved in mobilizing funding to address the needs of persons affected by the outbreak (Luce 2013). Further, as a city with a hub of healthcare organizations and academic healthcare research institutions including San Francisco General Hospital and University of California San Francisco Hospital, the city was also well positioned to generate more policy capacity in issues related to health and health services (H. Byrne 2018, Episode 6; Cisneros 2011; Luce 2013).

What the AIDS outbreak laid the groundwork for in homelessness policy was the development of a strong network of advocacy organizations, municipal public health infrastructure, and health clinics to treat displaced persons in need of medical care (Luce 2013, 146; W. Walker et al. 1997). Nearly 40% of persons with HIV/AIDS in San Francisco in the late 1980s were in need of housing (Mor et al. 1993). In response to the AIDS outbreak in the 1980s, the number of health clinics and advocacy organizations grew (Arno 1986; Blair 2016; Luce 2013). The City of San Francisco also increased the number of contracts with community organizations to provide services related to the AIDS outbreak (Arno and Hughes 1989; Morewitz 2018, 9;

W. Walker et al. 1997). University of California San Francisco Hospital and San Francisco General received increased federal funding from the Ryan White Care Act, the Centers for Disease Control and Prevention, and the City of San Francisco to invest in the outbreak response and in new homeless shelter construction, hospital beds, and behavioral health services (Arno and Hughes 1989; Blair 2016; Cisneros 2011; Luce 2013; Morewitz 2018, 31; W. Walker et al. 1997). The mayor during most of the outbreak, Art Agnos, ushered in extensive municipal investment in homeless shelters intended to transition to permanent housing for displaced and chronically homeless individuals (Fagan 2016; "Housing Beyond Shelter" 1990; Suzuki 2012).

The City of San Francisco established a municipal level AIDS office within the San Francisco Department of Public Health in 1985 (W. Walker et al. 1997). Additionally, the Department of Public Health increased funding to specifically provide services to individuals with HIV or those at risk of AIDS, with specific activities targeted to individuals in this group with co-occurring substance use disorders and a focused response targeting the psychiatric needs of HIV/AIDS patients (Blair 2016; Morewitz 2018, 9). This led to a direct municipal investment in behavioral health services for marginalized individuals with HIV/AIDS (McGarry 2008; Morewitz 2018; UC San Francisco Library Archives and Calisphere n.d.; W. Walker et al. 1997).

> So, it [the entity that started homeless policy efforts] was the Department of Public Health—it was the behavioral health providers, and the emergency system providers—so we operate the Sanctuary shelter that had been a bath house it opened post AIDS epidemic and the community is still thinking that this [AIDS] would be a long term problem.[5]

The archival records and extant literature demonstrate that the AIDS crisis, in particular, may have been the critical juncture by which San Francisco established vital policy capacity to respond to health crises for highly vulnerable groups. This influx of investment in healthcare, social services, and behavioral healthcare across the nonprofit sector, municipal government and healthcare organizations gave San Francisco the ability to address chronic illness when it arose as a salient policy issue beyond the HIV/AIDS epidemic. By the early 1990s, the substantial growth in local policy capacity to respond to the needs of vulnerable populations placed San Francisco in a position to respond to other similar issues, such as behavioral health and chronic homelessness, and transition to a greater municipal role in this policy space when the opportunity arose.

While San Francisco was adapting to a communicable disease crisis and mobilizing to establish sufficient medical and social service capacity to address the epidemic, the State of California was moving in a different direction on another very closely related issue: behavioral health.

There is a historical relationship between behavioral health and homelessness policy in the United States, aside from the relationship between severe mental illness (SMI) and long-term homelessness. When homelessness first arose as a national public policy topic in the 1980s, most researchers and policymakers saw rising rates of homelessness as directly related to deinstitutionalization in the 1960s or the closing of federal psychiatric institutions by the federal Community Mental Health Act (Prioleau 2013).

Media debates and federal bureaucratic debates (WHSOF Box 3 and Crippen 1987, 4; WHSOF Davis n.d., 2) assert that deinstitutionalization was the cause of the 1980s homelessness crisis in cities across the United States (Goldman and Morrissey 1985; Morrissey and Goldman 1984; Zlotnick, Zerger, and Wolfe 2013). In response, federal actors in the 1980s frequently highlighted deinstitutionalization as a rationale for *or* against decentralization of behavioral health services and homelessness programming, based on how actors attributed blame for the effects of deinstitutionalization (or its perceived relationship to rising rates of homelessness). For example, Republicans cited the failures of communities to effectively respond to deinstitutionalization by not creating community coordinated care and therefore promoting the homelessness of formerly institutionalized patients (WHORM File Box 43 1987). Democrats, on the other hand, cited the failure of the federal government to not fully implement/allocate funds to communities from the Community Mental Health Act ("National Homeless Awareness Week" 1986), therefore stifling programming and requiring a centralized, federal response to the homelessness crisis resulting from deinstitutionalization.

From this debate resulted the first and only federal law governing homelessness policy and programming. This law, the McKinney–Vento Act (now the HEARTH Act) (U.S. Department of Housing and Urban Development 2009), compromised between the two sides of the deinstitutionalization debate by establishing a federal law and federal regulations for homelessness funding and programming, while also establishing a decentralized network of "community" homelessness programming and decision-making, known as the federal Continuum of Care (CoC) (Davis Box 3 1987). McKinney–Vento set aside funds for homelessness programming but ultimately required cities to come together under the designated Continuum of Care structure to apply for federal funding to be used in homelessness programming (Jarpe, Mosely, and Smith 2019). This process is completely voluntary[6] and relies entirely on the Continuum of Cares to outline their individual needs and priorities, apply for funding, and organize and implement homelessness programming, typically without local governmental support (Jarpe, Mosley, and Smith 2019; Valero and Jang 2016).

California's entrance into the U.S. debate over the responsibility for persons affected by deinstitutionalization or persons with SMI (independent of homelessness) spoke directly to the policy cleavage between decentralized delivery of behavioral health services and programming or "community care," compared to recentralization or greater governmental participation, even if it wasn't the federal government itself taking responsibility (Vanneman and Snowden 2015, 593). Until 1990, California followed federal policy, decentralizing responsibility of behavioral health services, policy, and programming to communities or primarily nongovernmental actors, in regional community networks of care following deinstitutionalization under the Short–Doyle Act (Penner 1995, 275; Watson and Klurfeld 2011). California had followed federal policy based on the notion that community care was the most appropriate approach to mental illness and in the face of persistent concerns over the history of federal psychiatric care (Kennedy 1967). This decentralized model established entrenched community groups of primary nongovernmental actors with substantial expertise and capacity to deliver behavioral health services and programming (Aviram and Segal 1977; Penner 1995; Rochefort 1984; Zhang, Scheffler, and Snowden 2000).

Yet, in 1990, California was facing increasing budget challenges associated with community-based care and made the choice to reform this governance model (Masland 1996). During state-wide deinstitutionalization, the state of California had remained the administrative authority, although implementation was decentralized. In 1990, California chose to formalize administrative and funding provision for mental health services at the county level. While institutionally this was an act of administrative decentralization itself, the reform shifted control of policy implementation away from community-based organizations (CBOs) and directly to county governments. Instead of retaining the community networks of care, California reallocated governance authority from the networks of nongovernmental actors to counties (Penner 1995, 280; University of California Los Angeles n.d.).

This policy change was known as realignment. This shift occurred at the same time that the federal policy was enshrining the model of homelessness governance rooted in decentralization and community-based, voluntary programming. California chose to shift responsibility for behavioral health services to the county governments to improve tax and funding streams and better coordinate and standardize care (University of California Los Angeles n.d.)

For San Francisco and municipalities across California, realignment meant more responsibility for social and medical services serving persons with SMI would shift back to municipalities (R, A, and L 2001; Zhang, Scheffler, and Snowden 2000), as opposed to nongovernmental actors. As previously mentioned, in the federal debate—and, as we know today, for persons experiencing chronic homelessness—there is high overlap in populations targeted for behavioral health services for persons with SMI and homelessness programming for persons experiencing chronic homelessness. At the time in San Francisco, much of this population included individuals experiencing housing insecurity or homelessness after being diagnosed with HIV/AIDS (Arno 1986, 1326; City of San Francisco Department of Public Health 2000, 45; Mor et al. 1993).

The governance shift induced by realignment occurred right after San Francisco had already invested heavily in behavioral health infrastructure and policy capacity in response to the HIV/AIDS crisis (Blair 2016; Mor et al. 1993). In effect, realignment was not as challenging for San Francisco as it was for other municipalities across California that faced policy capacity and resource constraints, along with pushback from CBOs who had historically been delivering these services (Mor et al. 1993; Penner 1995). San Francisco did receive pushback from the CBO community, but experienced a more natural transition as a result of the strong political mobilization and investment in behavioral health at the municipal level during the AIDS crisis (Blair 2016). "Now the County is the main hub [for behavioral health services]; focusing on local system of care rather than decentralized; we have to maintain those relationships, we can't get rid of [the] CBO's; it's a partnership. . . . We always have to fashion these policies and procedures in conversation with providers."[7]

As discussed in the previous section, investment in health and social services during the AIDS outbreak included strong investment in housing, homeless shelters, and behavioral health services. Many persons with HIV/AIDS needed housing and supportive services as a result of displacement and trauma (Mor et al. 1993; San Francisco Department of Public Health HIV Seroepidemiology Surveillance Section 1998). Simultaneously, rates of homelessness were increasing in San Francisco as a result of the economic crisis (Fagan 2016). Realignment's shift to delegating full responsibility for behavioral health service governance to San Francisco city and county at the peak of the homeless crisis and in the midst of the HIV/AIDS crisis, along with the high overlap of needs across the populations (Mor et al. 1993, 197), raised questions about a similar, centralized municipal role to directly address homelessness.

Realignment and Political Mobilization—San Francisco's Supportive Housing Policy

After Realignment and following the AIDS outbreak, San Francisco continued to increase municipal level investments in homelessness and supportive housing, to address homelessness among persons affected by HIV/AIDS (San Francisco Department of Public Health 2006, 2019). By 1996, San Francisco had reconfigured its Continuum of Care, to establish a municipally governed coordinating board for the Continuum of Care, with a Housing First approach to chronic homelessness (Department of Homelessness and Supportive Housing and City and County of San Francisco 2019). Interviewees stated that realignment was an important part of developing San Francisco's municipal approach to chronic homelessness. Starting with behavioral health, the city gradually increased investment and recentralized responsibility to more effectively coordinate and fund the delivery of behavioral health services and supportive housing, along with other social services, to address chronic homelessness in the Bay Area (San Francisco Budget and Legislative Analyst's Office 2016).

In the 1990s, the Department of Public Health said,

> 'Well we have lots of people who are severely disabled, many [mental health] challenges and need lots of help . . . housing is healthcare, DPH needs to be in the housing business, this was embraced very much in the era of Housing First, embraced by DPH. . . . We will go into housing development, the supportive housing business'.[8]

Today, San Francisco has a new municipal Department of Housing and Supportive Services explicitly tasked with ending homelessness in the city. The department is organized around and delivers services through a permanent supportive housing and Housing First approach (San Francisco Budget and Legislative Analyst's Office 2016).

Now that we know why San Francisco has a supportive housing policy, we must investigate why San Francisco has a serious homelessness crisis, despite successful establishment of this municipal-level supportive housing policy. Centralizing the Continuum of Care in municipal government increased the policy opportunities for San Francisco municipal supportive housing policy efforts by providing the Continuum of Care the authority to design and execute municipal homeless policy (as San Francisco did with the adoption of their local level supportive housing policy approach). Interview and archival results demonstrate that San Francisco currently suffers from an implementation crisis arising from competing policy approaches that often directly contradict local regulatory policies. This implementation crisis and competing policy approaches originate in part from increasing participatory inequity at the local level. This inequity is a result of changing local demographics, fueling power of elite preferences over other, marginalized groups and policy target populations. The lack of coordination or perpetual conflict across policy approaches between local elites, the State of California, and the Continuum of Care, reduce policy opportunities for publicly funded policies. When public policies fail, economic elite's preferences are generally further promoted in an uncontested policy space (Elkin 2008), as is the case currently in San Francisco.

One of the key takeaways from the research is who participates in San Francisco homeless politics matters for policy outcomes—and who that is has changed significantly over the past two decades. Most of the research participants reflected on this change and what this change in participation meant for supportive housing policy and addressing chronic homelessness in San Francisco. The next section discusses the influence of changing demographics in San Francisco for homeless and supportive housing policymaking and participatory equity in San Francisco's political economy. Overall, San Francisco's increasing population homogeneity toward wealthy, white elites constrains the political participation of racial/ethnic minority groups, low-income individuals, and individuals who are currently homeless, formerly homeless, and or at-risk of homelessness.

Urban politics research demonstrates this common trend in housing policy across the United States, where the majority of participants in housing policy debates and anti-homeless policies are white homeowners as opposed to target populations (Einstein, Palmer, and Glick 2018; Robinson 2019; Trounstine 2019). In effect, persons who are most affected by San Francisco's homeless policies are not involved in policy decision-making processes.

This section considers the ways that San Francisco's population demographics have changed in recent decades to create this new political economy within the city. The majority of interviewees discussed the shifting population demographics as a cause for concern that they felt introduced majority biases in local decision-making while catalyzing the housing and homelessness crisis, itself. Archival analyses and extant literature support these results. As discussed, participatory inequity or increased majority bias here increases policy conflict, decreases coordination across policy spaces and reducing policy alternatives for evidence-based, publicly funded municipal supportive housing efforts.

One of the most common themes across all interviews was the influence of changing demographics within San Francisco on policy preferences about homelessness and homeless policy outcomes. The majority of interviewees, many of whom have worked in San Francisco homeless policy or practice for many years, described the simultaneous influx of wealthy, primarily white elites, with the exodus of many racial or ethnic minority groups from the city, as a key factor shaping rates of homelessness and homelessness debates.

> [The] new population of people that have moved into San Francisco . . . a very large portion of people, have . . . first of all the Black community left about 10 years ago, when rent went up, now rent has almost tripled almost 10 times the amount it was. Now it's a bunch of people from other states that have never experienced this type of mental illness or drug addiction or homelessness are up in arms that their 5 million dollar house has a homeless person in the eaves-way so you know our new San Franciscans are a big problem for our work.[9]

Until the 2000s, San Francisco was home to the Harlem of the West, known for icons and landmarks of Black culture (Fuller 2016). Yet, this has changed dramatically over time. Whereas, in 1976, 1 in 7 San Francisco residents was Black, today it is 1 in 20 (Fuller 2016; San Francisco Department of Planning 2018). The majority of current Black San Francisco residents are middle- or low-income, many living in public housing (City and County of San Francisco 2010, 2018, 2020; Fuller 2016). Directly associated with the shifting economy toward tech, increasing housing and real estate prices drove out Black communities and businesses, while also losing demand for Black businesses in San Francisco's changing culture (Hwang 2015). Today, Black residents still living in San Francisco struggle to protect their livelihoods and communities from tech developers and elite investors following the ongoing socioeconomic shift (Kwak 2018). The continually increasing cost of living threatens Black residents' quality of life. Many residents face food and housing insecurity and question their ability to remain in the city (Whittle et al. 2015). Twenty-one percent of Black residents in San Francisco in 2018 had been threatened with eviction within the past five years (San Francisco Department of Planning 2018, 54).

Latinx families are facing a similar trend as Black Americans in San Francisco. From the late 1990s through the present, San Francisco's Mission District, a historically Hispanic neighborhood, has been heavily gentrified (Mirabal 2009). Many Latinos were forced out of the Mission District and San Francisco as a result of increased housing prices, tech boom development, and limited protections for low- or middle-income families in local housing policies (Mirabal 2009). From 2000 to 2005, 10% of San Francisco's Latino population moved out of the city in response to rising housing prices (Mirabal 2009). In 2018, 24% of Latinos living in San Francisco had been threatened with eviction during the past five years (San Francisco Department of Planning 2018, 54). Today, many Latinos are remaining in the Bay Area but moving into surrounding counties or lower-income neighborhoods (Bowe 2015). While housing insecurity and homelessness are increasing in San Francisco, minorities and those affected by or are at risk of homelessness who would benefit from redistributive housing policies are being pushed out. As discussed, previous research has shown that homogenous areas, particularly white, pass more restrictive and less evidence-based redistributive housing and zoning policies (Bates and Santerre 1994; Trounstine 2020).

The Tech Boom—Influx of Wealthy, Highly Educated Elites

The accumulating wealth of one primary population demographic influences local political dynamics including competition over resources, political participation and lobbying influence. These relationships will be evaluated in greater depth in the following section. The majority of interviewees discussed the migration of wealthy individuals to San Francisco as a key factor in political processes shaping supportive housing and homeless policy outcomes. Additionally, interviewees discussed other, acute and long-term effects of wealth influx on the housing market and ultimately rates of homelessness.

Increasing housing instability Black and Latino residents face is driven by the influx of wealthy elites moving to San Francisco, many to work in the tech industry. San Francisco is now home to more billionaires per capita than any region on earth (Heller 2019). Since 2000, the population of San Francisco residents with income over 200% of the AMI increased by nearly 250% (San Francisco Department of Planning 2018, 30). Subsequently, the percentage of residents with over 200% of the AMI now accounts for nearly 30% of San Francisco's population, compared to only 9% in 1990 (San Francisco Department of Planning 2018, 30).This influx of elites in response to the tech demand, increased San Francisco's overall socioeconomic status, and the city's economic homogeneity (Heller 2019). This growing economic homogeneity has promoted socioeconomic disparities between elites and other, lower income groups (San Francisco Department of Planning 2018, 54). Higher incomes over the AMI are disproportionately white, whereas low-income groups are majority people of color (San Francisco Department of Planning 2018, 50). Homeless rates across adults and the elderly have increased over the last half-decade, in response to rising housing prices and stagnated growth of low-income and supportive housing units (Applied Survey Research 2017, 76; City and County of San Francisco 2018; San Francisco Department of Planning 2018). Overall, increased wealth/white homogeneity increases opposition to redistributive policies and evidence-based homeless policies while also constraining participation in political debates from persons who would benefit from these policies.

Multiple interviewees discussed the relationship between single-resident occupancy (SRO) housing units and tech entrepreneurs. Since the 1950s, in San Francisco, SROs have been primarily allocated as low-income rental units (McGarry 2008). These units provided housing for many low-income single adults and elderly occupants (San Francisco Department of Public Health 2006). In the wake of the tech boom, many single adults working in tech opted to rent SROs as a quick fix for cheaper housing, offering more money to landlords and pricing out current renters. As a result, many previous renters end up on the streets. "Another big trend is the loss of affordable housing . . . 5 to 6 years ago [was] when we first started hearing about Twitter employees renting out rooms in these SROs, basically saying folks were coming and saying all I need is a bed, $1,000 room."[10]

Downstream, the concentrated influx of wealthy elites led to a steep increase in housing prices (as previously discussed). Over the past decade housing prices in San Francisco grew over 400% (Rahaim et al. 2018, 26). Ultimately, this demographic shift influenced the exodus of less wealthy racial or ethnic minority groups out of San Francisco while promoting housing insecurity and homelessness within the city (Policy Link, Program for Environmental and Regional Equity, and University of Southern California 2015; San Francisco Department of Planning 2018).

Summary

The growing homogeneity of San Francisco's political economy may not seem to be a problem at face value. Democracies are based in majority opinion. However, democracies, as the next section discusses, are rooted in protecting political participation for minority group members so that *all* groups are able to participate in political processes and do not face tyranny of the majority where majority opinion obscures minority preferences and voices (G. W. Brown, McLean, and McMillan 2018). The next section will evaluate how the increasing homogeneity of San Francisco's political economy is stagnating minority group political participation and, in particular, participation by target populations in supportive housing policy, homeless policies overall, and homelessness prevention efforts. Obscuring minority group and target population participation from supportive housing policy debates is not only antidemocratic (Lerman and Weaver 2018; Michener 2016; Michener 2017b) but also creates inherent challenges for supportive housing efforts by increasing the probability that policies may not work to their intended goals due to information asymmetries about policy workability on the ground (Lillvis and Greer 2016; Willison 2017). Increased inequity in political participation enhances policy opportunities for elites and reduces publicly funded policy opportunities, by promoting of elite preferences that conflict with supportive housing policy goals and exacerbate implementation challenges for supportive housing policy.

PARTICIPATORY INEQUITY AND THE COMPETING PREFERENCES BETWEEN ECONOMIC ELITES AND BUREAUCRATS

This section focuses on the dynamics of political participation in San Francisco's political economy of homeless politics—or debates over policies affecting people experiencing chronic homelessness. This section in particular emphasizes the mechanisms of elite participation and what this means for overall participation by actors in decision-making to address chronic homelessness. The political economy evaluates the degrees to which certain actors are constrained, while others may have greater ability to participate in political decision-making, emphasizing the role of financial capital as a means to sway power dynamics and engender political privilege (Elkin 2008). The research identified two main types of political participation in homeless policy debates: informal and formal processes. This section evaluates how economic elites participate in local politics surrounding homelessness and what that means for participation overall in terms of constraints on certain groups or more power for others across these two types of political participation processes. Ultimately, inequitable participation dynamics exacerbate coordination challenges across the competing policies, increasing policy opportunities for local elites while decreasing policy opportunities for publicly funded, evidence-based municipal homeless policies as a result of the economic and political power of elites that dominate policy implementation processes.

The influence of the dynamics and composition of the political economy matters for participatory equity in democracies (i.e., the variable plurality of political participation). Do all actors have comparable ability to participate in debates? If such debates or spheres of participation are dominated by one group or another, this affects overall policy outcomes and may bias policy outcomes in favor of one group over another. When thinking about health equity or civic engagement, this relationship is particularly important for marginalized communities who inherently have less political capital and have been, historically, purposefully excluded from policy debates (Anoll 2018; Bridges 1999; R. Mickey 2015; Soss, Fording, and Schram 2011; Trounstine 2008). Thus, minority group absence from political debates or constraints against minority group participation shifts dynamics in decision-making toward other actors or elites in particular. Finally, there is a history of exclusion of target populations from public health policy debates or the absence of input from groups who are specifically affected by public health policies (Einstein, Palmer, and Glick 2018, 2019; Lillvis and Greer 2016).

This research finds that economic elites dominate debates over approaches or solutions to chronic homelessness in San Francisco across informal and formal types of political participation. This result may not be particularly surprising given San Francisco's demography. It is surprising, however, given the HUD (2014) mandate to increase community participation and the implications of a lack of participatory equity for health policy outcomes. The absence of minority and target group preferences in San Francisco homeless policy debates directly interferes with regulatory supportive housing policy by prioritizing elite preferences and obscuring the needs of low-income groups and persons experiencing or at risk of homelessness who are most affected by the policies in question. This participatory chasm perpetuates coordination challenges in supportive housing policy implementation, swaying policy goals toward elite preferences and limiting policy alternatives for municipal supportive housing efforts.

This first section describes "informal" means of political participation by different groups in the political economy and the overall degrees of participatory equity in the political economy as expressed by actors in the field. Informal means of participation are defined here as impromptu engagement with policy makers or service providers about homelessness policy and programming, outside of scheduled policy debates or votes. This definition does include formal *channels* of engagement—such as calling or writing to a municipal supervisor about concerns or policy opinions or calling or submitting requests through 311—San Francisco's local hotline, and now website, and phone application that allows residents to get information and submit complaints, concerns, or service requests to the City and County of San Francisco (2019).

The other main mechanism of informal participation as discussed by policy actors is police engagement. Residents frequently call the San Francisco Police Department (SFPD) to report concerns about homelessness or make policy or service requests. Police officers interact with persons experiencing homelessness regularly, and they themselves are now policy implementers, across different types of homelessness policies. Police interactions affect service delivery itself and service delivery strategies. Therefore, police officers often become the first point of engagement or first mode of participation over homeless programming preferences by San Francisco residents.

Interviewees expressed frequent public, informal engagement through these different types of channels to express concerns about homelessness in the city. All interviewees who discussed informal channels of policy participation only discussed participation by wealthy residents. The residents described were typically residents living in desirable neighborhoods, who participate through informal channels to issue complaints or concerns about homelessness. The primary goal of these complaints, as described by interviewees, is to request the removal of individuals experiencing homelessness from an area, generally related to the visibility of homelessness and the desire for it to not be evident in a resident's neighborhood.

Although the goal of participation is the same across these channels, both types of participation end in different results for local supportive housing policy, planning, and implementation. Informal, elite engagement through the police leads to direct, often acute police responses to homelessness that interrupt access to services for persons experiencing homelessness. Informal, elite engagement with elected officials interferes with regulators' duties to implement supportive housing policies, as elected officials directly pressure bureaucrats in response to elite requests to address homeless behaviors as opposed to long-term solutions to chronic homelessness. Often times, this interference in bureaucratic duties takes the form of direct orders to pursue other activities not aligned with existing regulation. Multiple channels of informal, elite engagement increase coordination challenges in local, publicly funded, evidence-based homeless policy implementation and policy opportunities for elites to target homeless behaviors through these mechanisms.

Informal Elite Engagement and Policing

All interviewees described frequent interactions between police and individuals experiencing homelessness, primarily individuals experiencing chronic homelessness. Compared to Atlanta and Shreveport, police engagement with individuals experiencing homelessness in San Francisco works very differently. In this regard, police in San Francisco are specifically trained to engage with individuals experiencing homelessness through a harm reduction approach. This means that police first respond by redirecting individuals to social services before responding with a criminal approach (Lazar 2017, 14). San Francisco also has a designated policing unit, the Homeless Outreach Team, known as the HOT team, that exists to address calls related to homelessness (Lazar 2017). This training and expert response infrastructure is a result of San Francisco's integrated municipal approach to chronic homelessness. The Continuum of Care has been managed through the municipal government since 1996 and has subsequently been able to coordinate and develop policies across municipal spaces through that authority (Department of Homelessness and Supportive Housing and City and County of San Francisco 2019).

Despite this strong institutional policy capacity to develop appropriate responses to chronic homelessness through policing, tension remains between elite preferences, the reality of chronic homelessness, and municipal, regulatory policy goals. This tension arises as a result of rising rates of chronic homelessness, resulting increased visibility of homelessness, and strong elite preferences that are further magnified through San Francisco's socioeconomically homogenous population.

> I think from the point of view of an average SF person, which is an extremely affluent city, the problem of homelessness is they don't like seeing people who look homeless, people who are racial minorities, people who are behaving in

ways that are unconventional, nonconformist, or just people who are hanging around outdoors.[11]

This tension comes to light when wealthy residents issue informal complaints, requests, concerns, or otherwise about individuals experiencing chronic homelessness through the SFPD.

The majority of interviewees, and all interviewees who responded to prompts about policing and homelessness, stated that citizens account for the majority of requests for police responses to homelessness in San Francisco. Interviewees also stated that complaints primarily arise from residents living in desirable or wealthy neighborhoods.

> People are very into their neighborhoods, quaint place with Victorian houses, density of houses is very difficult to build on 49 square miles, still single-family homes, no density . . . [opposition] is liberal, wealthy, etc. [They] don't want poor people living in their neighborhoods.[12]

> Here they are trying to fix a . . . great deal of frustration by SF residents, by what they term as "street behaviors," . . . so you have many highly visible people, some having bad street behaviors that are distressing to citizens of SF, who then call police or call 311.[13]

Municipal policing records were not available to measure the presence of citizen requests. However, publicly available 311 data were used to measure the frequency of requests (most 311 data includes police responses; City and County of San Francisco 2019). The 311 data concords with the interviewee results, demonstrating the very high frequency of 311 requests made about homelessness, especially behaviors associated with chronic homelessness. Homeless encampment cleanup was the third most common type of request made through 311 from 2008 to 2019, with 172,483 calls[14] or nearly 50 calls per day regarding encampments alone (not including other calls related to other behaviors associated with chronic homelessness; City and County of San Francisco 2019).

Some interviewees emphasized that not all requests for police responses to homelessness are negative. Interviewees stated that many are made out of genuine concern for individuals in these circumstances. The main theme interviewees reiterated was that regardless of the reason for requests for police responses, these responses often end in outcomes that contradict municipal, regulatory policy initiatives seeking to end chronic homelessness, detracting from local supportive housing policy efforts and reducing policy success.

Residents, in particular economic elite engagement through policing, have a direct and acute influence on local supportive housing policy and homeless policy outcomes. Interview results and 311 data demonstrate that when residents reach out to police regarding behaviors associated with homelessness, the responses often end in outcomes that conflict with supportive housing and Housing First policy goals. As shown in Figure 5.1, despite HOT Team protocol and training, individuals experiencing chronic homelessness are often fined, removed from an area and/or homeless encampments, and possessions are removed—five times more often than persons are referred to services or receive outreach.

In 2016, 70% of a survey of nearly 400 persons experiencing homelessness in San Francisco were forced from an area (University of California Berkeley School of Law Human Rights Center 2017). Sixty-nine percent received citations, and 22% received more than five citations (University of California Berkeley School of Law Human Rights Center 2017). While these police responses aligned with preferences about the desirability of homelessness, and possibly even public health concerns over sanitation and waste, redirecting individuals experiencing chronic homelessness into jail or away from certain areas creates barriers to supportive housing policy implementation by interfering with service engagement opportunities.

Just as in Atlanta and Shreveport, when individuals experiencing chronic homelessness are incarcerated, they are directed away from supportive housing prioritization efforts. Upon re-entry from jail, individuals are often not directed to social services (Hawthorne et al. 2012; Segal,

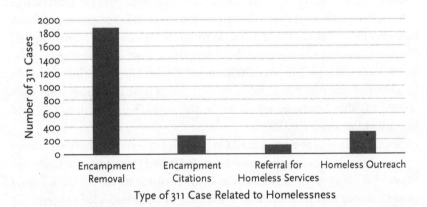

Figure 5.1 Responses to homelessness through 311 calls in San Francisco, 2009–2019. The data come from the publicly available San Francisco 311 data portal. Search terms to proxy measures of encampment removal, encampment citations, referral for homeless services, and homeless outreach in the database included "Homeless Encampment Remove," "Encampment Outreach," "Homeless Refer Referral Referred," and "Cited Encampment." The data presented include the total 311 case counts for each search query from 2009–2019.

Frasso, and Sisti 2018; Ware and Dennis 2013). As a result of this service gap, many individuals remain homeless upon re-entry and face challenges being redirected to points of service to mitigate homelessness and address behavioral and physical health issues (U.S. Department of Health and Human Services Assistant Secretary for Planning and Evaluation and Office of Disability Aging and Long-Term Care Policy 2018).

Relocating individuals experiencing chronic homelessness to different neighborhoods and/or destroying encampments has a similar outcome. Individuals are often moved to districts with fewer resources and/or further away from areas with social service points. In response, providers may have a harder time locating individuals and continuing outreach efforts.

> Right now there is a big effort to clean up the streets, get people living in tents off the streets, [they use the] sweeping the streets approach, they come and throw [homeless people's] stuff away to get them to move on, in theory they are supposed to have people linking them to services, but there aren't enough beds and no housing, so a lot of those people [homeless] are ending up in jail because of warrants or whatever.[15]

Overall, police responses to homeless behavior as a result of elite and citizen requests do not solve chronic homelessness and have the effect of continuously creating barriers to supportive housing policy implementation by restricting service access and engagement efforts resulting from conflicting policy goals (Mcnamara, Crawford, and Burns 2013; Roy et al. 2016).

Informal Elite Engagement and Elected Officials

This section demonstrates the tension and divergence between municipal regulatory decision-making and elite preferences in San Francisco homeless policy or policy conflict due to the separation of these two interests in their differing policy processes: the integrated municipal and Continuum of Care policy efforts and local economic elites. Overall, this research finds that regulatory decision-making is influenced by informal pressure from elected officials, and elected officials' behavior is shaped by economic elites. Suffice to say, San Francisco's responses to chronic homelessness from a regulatory perspective are swayed by typically short-term preferences of wealthy residents.

Beyond policing as an informal space for policy engagement, elected officials receive informal feedback from San Francisco residents about homeless policy efforts. The majority of interviewees described frequent communication between residents and elected city supervisors[16] about homelessness and chronic homelessness in San Francisco. Interviewees, similar to policing engagement discussions, described primarily wealthy residents as comprising the majority of informal lobbying efforts— emails, phone calls, etc.—to municipal supervisors about homelessness.[17] This included all interviewees working in the municipal bureaucracy and interviewees engaged as stakeholders in policy spaces and debates.

The informal policy engagement interviewees described works in similar ways as the engagement through policing but to a different end. Ultimately, informal, elite engagement with elected officials puts pressure on municipal bureaucrats, both indirectly and directly, to change supportive housing policy goals and implementation, away from evidence-based approaches and toward elite preferences prioritizing short-term outcomes addressing behaviors associated with homelessness.

A main theme that arose from interviews with municipal bureaucrats is the degree to which pressures from political actors—as a result of pressure from economic elites—impedes bureaucrats' ability to carry out work to their intended policy goals. Here, I define pressure on the bureaucracy as both direct pressure from elected officials on bureaucrats, as well as public pressure on elected officials that translates into action directed to, or pressure on, bureaucrats. The challenge arises here, as much of political science finds, in that bureaucrats are supposed to carry out purposes of legislation, or promulgate rules based on existing legislation, based on their expertise. If legislators are directly influencing bureaucrat's ability to carry out rules, the bureaucracy is not only politicized, but also policies may not work well to their intended goals or may not function well due to a lack of expertise to which the bureaucracy is central (Greer, Wismar, and Figueras 2016; Huber and Shipan 2002).

For public health, this tension or influence matters if elected officials' preferences conflict with evidence-based practices or cause harm by limiting bureaucrats' ability to implement such practices or policies. In interviews, municipal bureaucrats identified three main ways that elected officials responding to elite requests impeded pre-existing supportive housing policy goals: (1) pressure to act faster or at a pace that does not align with effective supportive housing policy implementation; (2) pressure to address homeless behaviors as opposed to identifying effective solutions to chronic homelessness; and (3) pressure against building new housing infrastructure for permanent supportive housing or low-income housing generally.

The first theme discussed by interviewees working in the municipal bureaucracy was the conflict between the pace or timing of supportive housing policy. Different notions about the desired pace of homeless solutions was a source of pressure for bureaucrats that manifested as a direct challenge to implementing intended municipal supportive housing policy goals.

Overall, bureaucrats stated that effective implementation of supportive housing policy required a careful, long-term approach to house individuals long term and end homelessness (San Francisco Budget and Legislative Analyst's Office 2016). Elites desire a short-term approach that typically does not align with evidence-based strategies and prefer to address homelessness as soon as possible (Takahashi 1997; University of California Berkeley School of Law Human Rights Center 2017). Interviewees emphasized that this latter preference is incompatible with the mechanisms required to implement permanent, supportive housing.

> The speed which certain things are done in the community and what is prioritized on a week by week basis may also be motivated by how the others in the neighborhood are experiencing people who are homeless in the neighborhood and encampments and encampment resolution team.[18]

All in all, elite informal engagement with local elected officials initiates informal policy processes that directly interfere with the regulatory goals of ongoing municipal supportive housing policy. In some instances, bureaucrats actually described their policy implementation processes and goals being changed immediately upon request or order from elected officials.

> There is a lot of . . . political power to clean things up quickly. . . . It looks like a mandate to take anyone from the San Francisco Police Department, who is using any substance on the street to take people off the street and bring them in, and it's over capacity to [our public clinic], there is no protocol to handle a totally different clinical protocol [e.g., different diagnoses] . . . [there is] opposition from our [clinicians] that there was a mandate that started yesterday, and we don't have the resources to do this, but opposition is not that they [clinicians] don't want to, but that we don't have the resources to do it. There is no name of the [new] mandate, you're probably gauging how I feel.[19]

A secondary theme discussed by interviewees in the municipal bureaucracy was pressure on bureaucrats from elected officials, stemming from elite requests to address homeless behaviors as opposed to identifying and implementing solutions to chronic homelessness, which is the intended goal of supportive housing policy. The context of this informal engagement is similar to the elite informal engagement with SFPD through requests to respond to behaviors associated with chronic homelessness. Here, interviewees stated that requests to address homeless behaviors were often made in response to public complaints about the visibility of persons experiencing chronic homelessness in their neighborhoods (of work or residence).

> We had the homeless response coordinated more around city districts, so each district would have a response team that knew homelessness in terms of relationships . . . so they knew the people to engage them in care. This was hard because even if that's your core job, you would still end of getting phone calls from constituents about specific homeless people, the Supervisor or Mayor would call and demand action, made it hard to be responsive in a meaningful way.[20]

Visibility of chronic homelessness may include simple prominence—persons experiencing chronic homelessness sitting, sleeping, etc. on sidewalks or walkways in neighborhoods or outside of offices. Visibility also includes the conspicuousness of injection drug use, public intoxication, and or behaviors associated with mental illness or psychosis in public areas.[21]

The main outcome interviewees described from this pressure on elected officials and then to bureaucrats is to institute a competing policy goal for bureaucrats: addressing behaviors associated with chronic homelessness as opposed to addressing the causes of chronic homelessness. The effect at the municipal level creates further fracturing within the municipal government that generates challenges for implementing effective, coordinated supportive housing policy.

> And mainly it's [cleaning up the streets approach] reactive to complaints by citizens—but in the process, it's not just a clear out of here approach, coupled with offering services; complicated because you move them [homeless] from one are, and they move to another. Mayors are definitely under pressure; city is under pressure for people who can't conceivably understand why the city is allowing these things [homeless behaviors] to happen.[22]

Interviewees gave multiple examples where elite pressure has led to regulatory changes or even additional homelessness programming that competes with or detracts from municipal Housing First efforts.

The primary example cited by the interviewees involved is the recent development of "Navigation Centers." Navigation Centers are "low-threshold, high-service residential programs for adults experiencing homelessness in San Francisco" (Department of Homelessness and Supportive Housing

2019b). Navigation Centers were introduced in 2015 in response to growing rates of chronic homelessness and are meant to increase shelter space while individuals transition to permanent housing options (Department of Homelessness and Supportive Housing 2019b). Many interviewees were frustrated by the Navigation Center initiatives because they do not address the causes of chronic homelessness.

> The city then turned towards emergency responses as opposed to prevention, the number of emergency shelter beds is very low in San Francisco, that's where they are focusing right now, this is inadequate because it reduces tension in the city to solve the problem. And all of these Navigation Centers are just shelters. Nothing special.[23]

Interviewees emphasized that while the Navigation Centers are not harmful, they take away resources that could be used for permanent supportive housing construction and ultimately focus more on reducing the visibility of homelessness in the short term, in line with elite preferences, without offering long-term solutions. Recent data from the Navigation Center outcomes to date show that half of clients in the Navigation Centers are discharged without permanent housing options (Birstow 2018; Department of Homelessness and Supportive Housing 2019a).

The new Incidence Command Structure (ICS), the system typically utilized for disaster responses in San Francisco has now been relegated to manage homelessness (Fracassa 2018). This change was another common example cited by interviewees, where elected officials introduced a change to regulatory approaches by treating chronic homelessness as an acute emergency response rather than an enduring problem necessitating long-term solutions.

> You would activate [ICS] in case of a disaster or catastrophe, earthquake, epidemic of something, . . . a sudden acute problem . . . activating this [ICS] for the problem of most chronic homeless in San Francisco, is at best somewhat perplexing, and reflects them reading into it, well what are, when you're going to fix homeless problem, what are you saying you're going to fix, here they are trying to fix a great deal of frustration by the police, and great deal of frustration by SF residents.[24]

Interviewees felt that pressure from residents to reduce the visibility of chronic homelessness was leading to a fracturing in the bureaucratic responses to homelessness in San Francisco by prioritizing shorter-term solutions that do not effectively end chronic homelessness (Eskenazi 2019).

The final theme that municipal bureaucrats discussed as pressure from elected officials comes in the form of a direct implementation challenge. Municipal bureaucrats are tasked with ending chronic homelessness—which requires housing individuals who are experiencing chronic homelessness and therefore requires housing infrastructure. However, municipal bureaucrats face constant backlash against new housing infrastructure. This includes pressure from the public/elected officials, cuts to plans or funding for new housing stock, or pushback against plans for additional housing stock. Even the Navigation Centers, although they are not housing, received significant public pushback despite their inception stemming from elite requests against homeless visibility (Birstow 2018, 3; Fracassa 2019a).

The pressure against building any type of new, low-income housing is a constant source of strain for bureaucrats because it inhibits them from solving the ultimate cause of homelessness—housing insecurity/access to affordable housing—as well as ending chronic homelessness, which requires access to permanent supportive housing units. Municipal bureaucrats described pressure against low-income housing as a persistent challenge that increased in recent years and inhibits implementing supportive housing policy goals. Bureaucrats frequently stated that they are limited in their ability to act, since shortage of low-income housing affects the ability to move forward with housing people and therefore ending chronic homelessness.

> San Francisco's goal is Housing First, but I think it's hard to achieve in a city where housing stock is so low. . . . People are making a lot of efforts to get people treated. . . . You know we can refer people to residential treatment, but we don't have any ability to get people into housing, and I think that's a very permanent experience that is very challenging for our patients.[25]

Elite engagement increased through these informal policy mechanisms in a space that is already typically biased toward elite preferences. Increased elite engagement through these informal policy mechanisms perpetuates a disjointed approach to chronic homelessness in San Francisco, with conflicting policy goals that undermine municipal policies and prioritize elite preferences for nonevidence-based approaches.

Formal Engagement

Formal political participation is the second type of political participation in homelessness politics in San Francisco. This includes participation scheduled specifically to initiate participation by different groups of actors. As opposed to the first type of participation, which requires initiative by citizen actors, this type of participation happens when policy makers schedule opportunities for the public to participate in policy debates in a formal setting or respond to proposed policies. This type of participation includes community meetings about homeless policy or development and solicited community input from the Continuum of Care in their Annual Action Plan. Federal HUD funding for the Continuum of Care since 2012 has required "community input" from the Continuum of Care during their planning processes to improve equity in these procedures (U.S. Department of Housing and Urban Development 2014).

The interviews and archival analyses demonstrate that as with the informal types of political participation, formal participation is concentrated by elites. This is in part due to the increasing homogeneity of San Francisco's demographics (influx of wealthy elites leading to rising housing prices and an exodus of lower income and minority communities) as previously discussed. This is also in part due to accessibility issues inherently facing low-income communities and at-risk populations. Individuals with lower income may have less time off from work to attend formal community meetings, face transportation challenges, etc. (Lucas 2012). Individuals experiencing or formerly homeless are often not represented at meetings for many reasons, including the reality that individuals at risk of or experiencing homelessness face greater acute needs weighted against formal political engagement.

> A challenge in policy promulgation is who's in the room from the community to give input—African American–led CBOs have trouble—another challenge is folks with lived experience being in the room sometimes difficult with how they are facilitated to give your input, lots of barriers to participating.[26]

The majority of interviewees described high participation in formal community meetings from wealthy residents on homeless policy and programming. Further, interviewees stated that the majority of the discussions or preferences cited at these meetings were related to complaints about the visibility of homelessness, behaviors associated with homelessness and SMI, and "not in my backyard" (NIMBY) preferences where wealthy residents emphasized that, regardless of the solutions on the table, the solution should not happen near their place of work or residence.

> There is a lot of [economic] change in the city—different stakeholder groups and different residents that have very different opinions—public safety

meetings—people who come and have a bone to pick—crazy ideas about how homeless people are bringing crime—the public seems to be very split—often split along class lines. . . . [People say,] "We just need law and order, put them in jail, criminalize them for continuing to show up in front of my house."[27]

Most interviewees described that individuals at risk of homelessness, formerly homeless or currently homeless almost never attend community meetings and or have opportunities to speak if they do attend.

Community input has been quite weak, [the] voice of people experiencing homelessness has been exceptionally weak in that [Continuum of Care implementation] process, it definitely feels like a sort of . . . yeah, we have to do this that gets us [federal] funding, but it's not where the policy making action is, it's not where the activity is.[28]

The majority of interviewees described that this pressure from wealthy residents in formal community debates is one of the greatest barriers to supportive housing policy implementation (Birstow 2018). The most common barrier cited aligns with the discussion in the previous section regarding implementation. Interviewees emphasized strong opposition to new housing construction. Interviewees elucidated that this barrier to housing construction directly inhibits supportive housing policy implementation goals. Even though San Francisco approaches chronic homelessness through a Housing First approach, it is ineffective unless there are housing units available to provide to clients.

NIMBYISM is incredible, no one can build but no one wants it . . . that population with severe meth psychosis are really struggling; then people are aging, more disabilities, and then they become homeless and they have a disability and there is no place to go. [29]

The current state of formal political engagement and the existing barriers for minority and target population participation in formal debates promotes participatory inequity in San Francisco's political economy. It might seem reasonable to say that participatory inequity doesn't matter if the existing political participation is representative of the current municipal demographics. However, San Francisco's changing political economy was instigated through the housing crisis. Today, San Francisco's demographics are not totally homogenous, and democratic political participation must include and protect minority group participation (Grogan and Park 2017; Michener 2017). Further, San Francisco's homeless population is growing: 2019 estimates counted 9,808 individuals experiencing home-lessness in the City of San Francisco (City and County of San Francisco 2019). The risk of perpetuating participatory inequity in San Francisco's po-litical economy is to obscure minority populations' voices and preferences and the preferences and voices of individuals who are targeted by the policies under debate: policies affecting individuals experiencing or at risk of homelessness and chronic homelessness. Constraining political partici-pation by affected or targeted populations may undermine policy effective-ness (Lillvis and Greer 2016).

In time, the continued inequity in San Francisco's political economy may actually perpetuate the homelessness crisis by eliminating input from af-fected populations and thus tailoring policy solutions to elite preferences aimed at homeless behaviors instead of long-term solutions to chronic homelessness. This outcome is not preferred by any group. The lack of co-ordinated policy solutions as a result of conflicting policy approaches be-tween elites and local government, exacerbated by political participatory inequity, reduces policy opportunities for municipal supportive housing policies and increases policy alternatives aligned with elite preferences.

Summary

This section shows that participatory constraints on pluralistic, democratic participation may be inhibiting the elite and the integrated Continuum of Care and municipal government from aligning and coordinating across policy spaces. San Francisco's political economy is one where economic elites dominate public debates over homeless policy, with the absence of marginalized populations and groups directly affected or targeted by these policies: persons experiencing homelessness or formerly homeless and persons at risk of homelessness. These divergent policy processes with competing policy goals reinforce participatory inequity by offering mul-tiple, concurrent channels of participation dominated by elites while also generating regulatory hurdles and implementation challenges for local supportive housing efforts that detract from original supportive housing policy goals and hinder success.

Without improving participatory equity, the outcome for homeless policy implementation may remain skewed toward policies favoring eco-nomic elites and that do not directly address homelessness, perpetuating policies in direct conflict with policies pursued by the city of San Francisco addressing the causes of chronic homelessness. This participatory eq-uity also bleeds into the influence of elected officials on the bureaucracy.

Elected officials create tension and conflict for pre-existing policies seeking to mitigate chronic homelessness, by constantly attempting to restructure policies and shift them from their intended goals (Pierson 1993), creating barriers and challenges to service delivery and implementation. As these processes continue, bifurcating policy mechanisms and goals, viable policy opportunities for local supportive housing efforts may continue to decline or stagnate.

BRINGING THE STATE BACK IN

The State of California acts as another, perhaps unexpected, conflicting actor or source of competing policies with divergent goals, design, and implementation mechanisms compared to the policies targeting chronic homelessness on the ground in San Francisco through the municipal Continuum of Care. The state-level policies seek to address homelessness in different ways compared to municipal approaches, and coordination with municipal approaches is limited. The competing policies and politics stemming from California's state-level policies act as direct and indirect barriers to municipal supportive housing policy design and implementation in San Francisco. These competing policies facilitate barriers to local efforts by generating administrative burden (Moynihan, Herd, Rigby 2016) and funding constraints that inhibit local supportive housing efforts and reduce successful municipal supportive housing policy implementation.

As reflected in the interviews, the State of California exists as a primarily separate governance structure with independent decision-making and implementation processes. California has many policies with the potential to assist supportive housing efforts and reduce chronic homelessness. However, the majority of existing state-level policies have not been fully implemented, leading to resource constraints. Alternatively, the policies work across different assumptions about population needs, creating administrative barriers for local policy efforts. All in all, these state policies fall short for homeless providers and individuals experiencing chronic homelessness in San Francisco as a result of divergent policy goals and policy processes. Responding to the existing challenges with state level policies, the majority of interviewees said that the state isn't doing much and could be doing more.

Interviewees and archival analyses identified two main policies encompassing state policies affecting or intended to manage chronic homelessness in California. These policies are (1) Medicaid and (2) the millionaires tax. A third policy space was mentioned tangentially, the California

Interagency Council on Homelessness. The majority of interviewees did not mention the California Interagency Council on Homelessness, and the interviewees who did only mentioned it to say that they were not aware of anything that the agency had done. Therefore, the California Interagency Council on Homelessness was omitted from the results due to limited salience among local policymakers. There are other policies that address other issues associated with chronic homelessness that did not arise as primary concerns for interviewees. These and other policies (e.g., Conservatorships, Community Development Block Grant and Supplemental Nutrition Assistance Program funding) may be a part of the existing state policy space but are not reviewed here due to their limited salience among policy makers at the local level.

Interview and archival analyses revealed two primary challenges from the state level policy space that conflict with or directly impede local level supportive housing policy making and implementation: (1) conflicting policy goals and (2) implementation challenges—defined here as administrative burdens and funding challenges. Based on the results, implementation challenges appear to come from conflicting policy goals. The reduced coordination between state and local policies ending in conflicting goals and administrative burdens further restrict successful policy opportunities for local supportive housing policy efforts.

Medicaid and Conflicting Policy Realities

As discussed, the health effects of homelessness are immense, increasing mortality, rates of chronic and communicable diseases, and adverse behavioral health outcomes including SMI and substance use disorders (Fazel, Geddes, and Kushel 2014; Maqbool, Viveiros, and Ault 2015; Stringfellow et al. 2016; Young and Manion 2017). The acute and long-term health consequences of homelessness most often require access to health services as well as housing (U.S. Department of Housing and Urban Development 2016; Kertesz et al. 2016). This dual approach has been shown to lessen homelessness, reduce morbidity and mortality, and improve quality of life (Doran, Misa, and Shah 2013; Larimer et al. 2009; U.S. Department of Health and Human Services Assistant Secretary for Planning and Evaluation and Office of Disability Aging and Long-Term Care Policy 2014). Before the Affordable Care Act, many homeless adults, primarily single men, did not have health insurance coverage. Lack of health insurance limited the scope of services and programming that could be offered to address homelessness and improve health outcomes. In the wake of the Affordable

Care Act, many practitioners and advocates hoped that Medicaid expansion would substantially improve access to necessary supportive medical services to more effectively address the complex medical conditions many homeless patients face (Tsai et al. 2013).

Interview results demonstrate that Medicaid expansion did not significantly influence municipal homelessness policy functioning due to divergent policy goals between state and local policy, resulting in two types of implementation challenges: (1) administrative burdens and (2) funding limitations. A lack of an influence of Medicaid expansion on San Francisco's municipal homeless policy is surprising, because many policy makers viewed Medicaid expansion as a kind silver bullet, anticipated to greatly improve access to healthcare for persons experiencing all types of homelessness, in particular individuals experiencing chronic homelessness. These implementation challenges interfere with municipal supportive housing policy implementation, creating further challenges for successful local policy opportunities.

Divergent Policy Goals

The divergent goals between municipal regulatory supportive housing policy and California's Medicaid expansion are not difficult to see. San Francisco's supportive housing policy is targeted directly toward individuals experiencing chronic homelessness and focuses on addressing the causes of homelessness through access to housing, medical/behavioral, and social services. Medicaid expansion was never intended to specifically target individuals experiencing homelessness. Medicaid as a policy focuses solely on providing healthcare insurance coverage to low-income individuals and low-income persons with disabilities. There is a clear overlap in populations served by the two policies. However, the goals of the policies are so different that the population of interest—in this case persons experiencing chronic homelessness—interact with two separate policies, in different ways, and to different ends.

Supportive housing policy is designed to explicitly address the needs of this high-risk population. Medicaid expansion serves a large and relatively diverse population and therefore does not have population specific policy goals or implementation mechanisms (beyond retaining categories of able bodied or not; Grogan, Singer, and Jones 2017). At face value, this may not seem to be a challenge and is perhaps a virtue of Medicaid by not differentiating coverage across social categories. Yet, where state and local policy goals engender policy conflict, the fact is that homelessness programming relies on and in many cases requires Medicaid as a major payer of medical services that are used in homelessness programming and supportive housing (Cassidy 2016). Therefore, if Medicaid policy works on different priors of access and eligibility not aligned with needs specific to persons experiencing homelessness or long-term homelessness, Medicaid creates unintentional access barriers and challenges for homeless policy and programming implementation. This dysfunction emphasizes the importance of coordination—especially in distinct systems where one has been built to rely on the other. Alternatively, if coordination is not possible, the challenges inhibiting policy success bring into question whether or not Medicaid is an adequate support policy.

Implementation Challenges—Administrative Burden and Funding

Medicaid's goal to expand insurance access for recipients is vital for supportive housing policy. This focus on coverage access is also where the Medicaid policy processes begins to diverge from homelessness policy goals by generating administrative burden inhibiting access to Medicaid for individuals experiencing homelessness and chronic homelessness.

The traditional methods of distributing access to Medicaid do not translate directly to persons experiencing homelessness. In California, the state is the main administering entity for Medicaid and sets policies for eligibility and enrollment (Department of Health Care Services State of California 2019b). Yet, under state administration, many eligibility determinations and program implementations are designated to local county welfare offices (Department of Health Care Services State of California 2011; Department of Health Care Services State of California 2019a).

Interviewees described that county-level administration increases administrative burden on enrollees who are homeless by requiring residency in the county of enrollment and tying enrollment to residency. Most persons experiencing homelessness, particularly chronic homelessness, do not have an address by virtue of being homeless. Individuals who are chronically homeless often move in and out of county lines for service utilization (Degeorge 2010; Gray et al. 2011; Metraux, Treglia, and O'Toole 2016). Both factors increase disenrollment, or enrollment churning, for persons experiencing homelessness (Sommers et al. 2016; State Health Access Data Assistance Center, Division of Health Policy and Management, and University of Minnesota School of Public Health 2018). Interviewees outlined the challenges associated with Medicaid enrollment and how it has not worked as well as anticipated for retaining healthcare coverage and improving access to necessary health services as a result of administrative burden.

> Oh yes—Medicaid expansion means that most of the homeless people are basi-cally eligible for Medicaid, our biggest issue is Medicaid retention—terminating enrollment is a huge issue—the homeless people don't fill out the paper work and get kicked off . . . a few people move out of County—all of Medicaid in California is county based—which doesn't make sense with cities. Homeless people travel around the state and hop around. Your Medicaid benefits are tied to the county you live in, so when you show up, if you're trying to get them into the behavioral health system, you have to track down what their residence is, or the county pays for it out of their budget.[30]

Medicaid implementation challenges resulting from administrative burdens also intersect with the existing challenges in the crowded policy space surrounding chronic homelessness. High rates of incarceration among individuals experiencing chronic homelessness (Hawthorne et al. 2012; Tsai and Rosenheck 2012; Volk et al. 2016)—as a product of reac-tionary policing responses most often pushed by economic elites to address homeless behaviors as previously discussed—create inherent challenges for Medicaid eligibility.

Individuals previously enrolled in Medicaid are disenrolled when incarcerated and face re-enrollment barriers after being discharged (U.S. Department of Health and Human Services Assistant Secretary for Planning and Evaluation and Office of Disability Aging and Long-Term Care Policy 2018). Re-enrollment barriers stem from a lack of alignment with Medicaid administration and the carceral state. Many individuals who experienced homelessness prior to incarceration face a dearth of services and limited connections to services after re-entry, upon which many are released to homelessness (Snyder 2016a; U.S. Department of Health and Human Services Assistant Secretary for Planning and Evaluation and Office of Disability Aging and Long-Term Care Policy 2018). Very similar to results in Shreveport (see Chapter 7, this volume), the majority of interviewees in San Francisco cited that a lack of coordination between state Medicaid programming, local carceral policy, and municipal bureaucrats in the Continuum of Care promotes gaps in services upon re-entry and facilitates cycling of incarceration for individuals experiencing chronic homelessness.

> The problem is once you go into jail, this is all general funded no Medicaid in jail – so we can't afford certain things without grant funded programs. At the

same time, the people are here, they are at risk when they get released from jail.[31]

The misalignment of policy goals across state and local policies and policy processes further intensifies the administrative burden on individuals seeking services by placing enrollment responsibility on at-risk individuals, rather than supported enrollment relying on systems to catch vulnerable individuals. For persons experiencing chronic homelessness, who face higher rates of chronic medical conditions, disability, and high rates of SMI, stable access to medical services through continuous health insurance enrollment is crucial for supportive housing policy success and ending homelessness.

> The mental health system and substance use disorders system is episodic, you leave or get thrown out, discharged, and there are no services that are lifetime . . . when they [homeless] are discharged, there are no CBOs that are in charge of following a person through the process. That is what we [new Whole Person Care (WPC) Medicaid Waiver Program[32]] are trying to address. There is no such service [for coordination] . . . and you don't transition from one place to the next.[33]

Funding is the second means by which Medicaid goals are not aligned with supportive housing policy efforts, creating conflict and tension between the two policy initiatives. Divergent policy goals lead to increased policy conflict, arising in funding challenges. Medicaid funding statutorily cannot pay for housing (rent, housing construction, housing subsidies etc.; Paradise and Cohen Ross 2017). This barrier has been understood for a long time, and yet the effects of this policy conflict have not been well understood or examined. This funding constraint may not seem to be a direct policy conflict at first look. However, as mentioned Medicaid is the primary payer for wrap around supportive medical services for individuals experiencing chronic homelessness (Cassidy 2016). When Medicaid funds a large part of supportive housing policy implementation but not the majority, it not only creates funding challenges by producing complicated funding streams for supportive housing policies; it also raises the question of what role Medicaid should have in supportive housing and homeless policy.

> Medicaid through series of waivers in CA have allowed Medicaid to be used for wrap around funding—more savvy players are trying to use Medicaid to fund

services delivery part of [supportive housing], but it can't pay for brick and mortar, maybe in assisted living, [it] mostly its payed for wrap around services.[34]

The majority of interviewees cited Medicaid funding as a barrier to supportive housing implementation. This funding challenge acts as a persistent barrier to policy coordination across Medicaid and homelessness policy due to divergent policy goals. Interviewees stated that they face constant challenges as a result of policy complexity and funding gaps. HUD funding has not kept up with inflation and low-income housing needs over the past 10 years and has recently faced more cuts to low-income housing assistance (Mazzara 2018; Urban Institute and Kingsley 2017). Medicaid funding has increased and offers more opportunities for supportive medical services. Therefore, interviewees cited that local providers and policy makers face a trade-off where they may be able to provide medical services but have substantial gaps in funding to pay for housing. Medical services without permanent housing do not solve chronic homelessness and have been shown to be ineffective in ending homelessness alone. Both housing and medical care are required in tandem to end chronic homelessness (Leff et al. 2009). Medicaid's inability to pay for brick and mortar creates a perverse incentive where policy makers are able to spend more money on downstream services absent a vital upstream component necessary to end homelessness—housing. This perverse incentive emphasizing approaches to homelessness without housing is exacerbated by San Francisco's political economy prioritizing short-term solutions and actively pushing back against housing opportunities.

In the end, interviewees detailed that they face funding gaps, are unable to fully implement policies by prioritizing wrap around services without housing, and/or pursue multiple funding streams and face further administrative barriers when attempting to enact and implement policies that are funded through different pots of money and different funding requirements.

> [We work] to create the political role to create this [supportive housing policy] change, and to have the resources to do this . . . that the San Francisco Board of Supervisors understands . . . the funding we need at a local and state level to meet our goals. . . . The biggest challenge is having the funding in order to execute the plan. And we're not going to get it from the feds.[35]

Limited coordination between Medicaid expansion and local policy creates (1) implementation challenges ending in administrative burdens that reduce policy success on the ground and (2) funding challenges generating perverse incentives to prioritize supportive services over comprehensive supportive housing, in an already fragmented policy space that actively restricts homeless housing opportunities.

California's Mental Health Services Act, Policy Misalignment and Stagnation

The second policy area most often referenced in interviews and archival analyses and highlighted by the majority of interviewees as a policy space that created simultaneous hope for local policy initiatives and direct barriers to local supportive housing policy implementation, is the California Mental Health Services Act (MHSA). The MHSA was originally passed in November 2004. Alternatively known as the "millionaires tax," the act was intended to impose a 1% income tax on personal income in excess of $1 million to generate funding specifically designated for county-level behavioral health services (Department of Health Care Services State of California 2020).

Since its inception, the MHSA has suffered from both inconsistent policy goals and implementation problems. Although originally intended to support behavioral health service efforts at the county level, the policy was reconceptualized, and monies were promised to instead fund permanent supportive housing efforts. In both cases, the policies were never fully implemented, and funding has not been distributed as intended. Ultimately, the MHSA generated barriers to supportive housing policy implementation in San Francisco and across California by stagnating funding for permanent supportive housing construction originally intended to address high rates of chronic homelessness (The Editorial Board 2018).

The Mental Health Services Act's Evolution Toward New Policy Goals and Implementation Failures

Interviewees stated and archival research demonstrate that the MHSA evolved over time, shifting from the original policy and original policy goals. The initial MHSA taxed millionaires to gain revenue for behavioral health services at the county level, including but not limited to prevention services and community services and supports (Scheffler and Adams 2005). The MHSA has been collecting revenue since 2005, accumulating a total of $14.6 billion to date (California Mental Health Services Oversight and Accountability Commission 2019). Since then, MHSA has provided significant revenue to county-level behavioral health agencies, providing, on average, about one fourth of funding for county-level behavioral health services across California (County Behavioral Health Director's Association 2015). MHSA also has a target population focus specifically on SMI as opposed to targeting behavioral health services broadly across populations (County Behavioral Health Director's Association 2015). This shift to focus solely on SMI was hailed by stakeholders in homelessness programming and policy due to increases in chronic homelessness and unaddressed SMI needs for this population (San Francisco Department of Public Health 2019, 7).

The major policy shift happened in 2016 when then-Governor Jerry Brown instituted No Place Like Home (NPLH; California Department of Housing and Community Development 2019). NPLH was established to use MHSA money to specifically create new permanent supportive housing beds. NPLH would provide state-level bonds to providers to construct new permanent supportive housing units. The bonds would be repaid through the MHSA tax (California Department of Housing and Community Development 2019). While Continuum of Care providers across California and the municipal Continuum of Care in San Francisco were happy about this redirection of MHSA funding, many behavioral health providers were not. Some California providers felt that this funding should remain targeted at behavioral health services, especially in lieu of a severe psychiatric bed shortage across the state (White 2018; Witkin and Huang 2018). This policy shift created a fragmentation across the two stakeholder coalitions and pushback against MHSA's funding for supportive housing efforts.

The pushback from behavioral health coalitions was compounded by opposition from elites who, as discussed, continued to strongly oppose permanent supportive housing construction (Fracassa 2019b; Monkkonen and Livesley-O'Neill 2017; Waxmann 2019). Lobbying efforts from elites and behavioral health providers led to stagnated implementation of NPLH (Witkin and Huang 2018). Interviewees emphasized that they had not received any support from the state from NPLH, and this revenue loss has been a barrier to local supportive housing efforts in San Francisco. "No Place Like Home. . . . it's a state program that's meant to give counties funding for housing for homelessness. It's not established, maybe not even implemented."[36]

Similar to the absence of Medicaid dollars for permanent supportive housing, the retraction of promised NPLH funding for permanent supportive housing created intractable trade-offs in municipal supportive housing policy. First, the stymied funding for housing led local providers in San Francisco to not trust state-level supportive housing efforts and rely almost entirely on local funding initiatives. While San Francisco is able to leverage local funding, many localities do not have sufficient resources. In these cases, state-level policy failures may have a much more dramatic influence on local-level supportive housing and homeless policy efforts.

The absence of state funding further constrains local funding initiatives in an already limited local resource environment with severe policy capacity needs to address the homeless epidemic (San Francisco Budget and Legislative Analyst's Office 2016). By 2018, NPLH had not provided any monies for permanent supportive housing construction as a result of implementation challenges (L. Dillon 2018).[37] Lastly, the perverse incentives created by Medicaid promoting supportive services over housing, paired with the loss of permanent supportive housing funds from the MHSA, further reduce opportunities for funding housing to effectively end chronic homelessness, incentivizing money for downstream services in isolation. The reduced coordination or misalignment across policy spaces further hampers municipal supportive housing policy efforts and reduces policy opportunities for upstream, evidence-based policies.

The MHSA is different from Medicaid politics because it is an example where the conflict between policy goals led to complete policy implementation stagnation and, eventually, an inability of the state to fulfill its intended policy goals. The way that the policy goals and intentions changed over time created challenges for supportive housing policy by pursuing two very different policy outcomes—first behavioral health then supportive housing—and producing neither. The stymied implementation of NPLH ended with no permanent supportive housing units and ultimately reduced behavioral health funding. Each original policy goal spoke to different stakeholder communities. The shifting policy trajectories generated animosity among both stakeholder groups by not delivering the intended policy products.

Simultaneously, each policy trajectory also drew contingents of detractors—primarily from wealthy elites (Scheffler and Adams 2005). The shifting trajectories compounded with the failed implementation of state-level funding initiatives for permanent supportive housing under MSHA furthered animosity among detractors by providing rationales to repeal MHSA (Enos 2018). Overall, the modified policy trajectories ending in unattained policy goals created additional barriers to municipal supportive housing policy efforts by strengthening coalitions of elites who oppose supportive housing efforts and the original taxation, while also generating conflict and fragmentation among coalitions of behavioral health stakeholders and supportive housing stakeholders due to the failed implementation of both intended policy outcomes (Graves 2018; White

2018). The limited coordination between state policies targeting homelessness and local needs or policies on the ground ultimately reduced municipal evidence-based policy opportunities and increased opportunities for elites by further incentivizing short-term solutions.

Summary

The results of this section demonstrate the existence of separate policy processes between state and local policy regarding the goals policies seek to accomplish, the needs of targeted populations, and/or the processes used to accomplish these goals. This separation primarily arises from conflicting goals between local policymakers in the San Francisco Continuum of Care or municipal bureaucracy, and the State of California. Conflict is crucial to the success of democracies. Challenges arise and policies stagnate when conflict never subsides to overcome collective action problems and contributes to policy fragmentation affecting successful implementation. Here, the rift or divergence between local and state bureaucrats generated barriers for local supportive housing policy implementation. These policy misalignments not only influence the success of both state and local policy efforts, but also negatively influence the health and well-being of individuals experiencing chronic homelessness by constraining supportive housing policy implementation success and subsequently restricting access to critical medical services and supportive housing efforts.

SUMMARY

San Francisco illustrates the significance of policy implementation as a crucial process that cannot be overlooked when examining the success of policy initiatives. At first glance, San Francisco should be very well positioned to successfully tackle chronic homelessness compared to other cities across the United States. San Francisco has a strong municipal tax base that allows for local investments in social services that other municipalities are not able to provide. The liberal ideology of San Francisco historically placed the city on the forefront of innovatively tackling social problems related to chronic homelessness including HIV/AIDS and county-level behavioral health services. Finally, San Francisco has a municipally governed Continuum of Care that is supported by other strong, local social and health service programs including the Department of Public Health and the Human Services Agency. This position in local government granted San Francisco's Continuum of Care improved ability to participate in municipal decision-making related to homelessness and provided the Continuum of Care with authority to successfully design and carryout local policies related to homelessness. This is an advantage compared to other more decentralized, nongovernmental counterparts across the United States that have little to no governing authority and are limited in their ability to coordinate with police, county public health agencies, or elected officials or have little voice regarding municipal funding, zoning, or budget priorities.

Yet, despite these facets that would appear to place San Francisco at the pinnacle of success for supportive housing policy implementation, many of the Continuum of Care's efforts have been stagnated at the implementation phase as a result of elite interference and state-level administrative and funding constraints. Elites dominate San Francisco policy debates related to chronic homelessness, both formally and informally. In formal participation, elites overshadow municipal debates, and individuals affected by the policies in question are rarely present. The strength of elite preferences is magnified through multiple available informal channels of participation. Elites assert their preferences through these alternative policy mechanisms including policing and pressure on elected officials to intervene in undesirable regulatory policies or, in this case, supportive housing policy. HUD requires community participation in Continuum of Care planning processes. Yet, as this research illustrates, these processes are not equitable, and elite opinion overshadows the preferences of minority groups and individuals directly affected by homelessness programming and supportive housing policy, while simultaneously redirecting policy goals away from best practices to reduce chronic homelessness.

The State of California remains relatively separate from municipal activity attempting to mitigate chronic homelessness. State-level goals, including Medicaid and the MHSA, are not aligned with local supportive housing goals and are not tailored to address the needs of persons experiencing or at risk of homelessness and chronic homelessness. As a result, both state-level policies generate barriers for supportive housing implementation by establishing administrative burden to accessing health services for individuals experiencing chronic homelessness and restricting valuable funding streams to finance local supportive housing initiatives.

San Francisco is a city with a very visible homeless epidemic. The problem will not be solved until implementation problems can be overcome by improving participatory equity in political decision-making to include minorities and at-risk groups, limiting elected officials' ability to interfere with bureaucrats' duties to carryout supportive housing regulation, and improving state level coordination with municipal goals to reduce administrative burdens and potentially align funding mechanisms. All in all, until the fragmentation across the separate policy spaces can be reduced to eliminate conflicting policy goals, San Francisco will continue to exist in a constant state of failed policy implementation.

CHAPTER 6

The Fragmented State

Atlanta and the Challenges of Coordination

WHAT'S HAPPENING IN ATLANTA?

Atlanta, like San Francisco, has an integrated homeless governance system that is a part of municipal government and coordinates with other relevant municipal offices to promote evidence-based, municipal supportive housing policy efforts. These developments allowed Atlanta to make notable progress in reducing homelessness in the city in recent years and also to take action to reduce criminalization policing responses to homelessness. Yet, despite this success, Atlanta faces ongoing challenges regarding municipal supportive housing policy implementation. This chapter focuses on explaining why Atlanta still faces these significant challenges in policy implementation and decision-making regarding approaches to chronic homelessness. These challenges primarily include (1) jurisdictional boundaries affecting service delivery and responsibility, (2) economic elites and policing, and (3) funding and relationships between the State of Georgia and municipal entities. These ongoing challenges create a fragmented policy space similar to that in San Francisco, where multiple disjointed policy approaches with conflicting policy goals inhibit the success of municipal supportive housing policy implementation. Simultaneously, municipal institutional arrangements create havens of political decision-making that favor economic elites, increasing policy opportunities for private actors that conflict with evidence-based policy solutions, primarily through reactionary policing.

Ungoverned and Out of Sight. Charley E. Willison, Oxford University Press (2021). © Oxford University Press.
DOI: 10.1093/oso/9780197548325.003.0006

Atlanta is a large city in northwestern Georgia, with about half a million residents (Data USA 2020a). The poverty rate in the Atlanta metropolitan area in 2020 was nearly twice the national average at 22.4%. The majority of Atlanta's population identifies as Black (50.7%); 38 percent identify as white and less than 4% as Hispanic/Latino or Asian (Data USA 2020a). According to the U.S. Department of Housing and Urban Development (HUD), 4,317 persons were experiencing homelessness in the city Atlanta (not including overlapping counties) in 2015 (HUD 2015d). In 2018, that figure was 3,076 (HUD 2018d). Atlanta's overlapping counties of Fulton and DeKalb also reported reductions in homelessness between 2015 and 2018 (HUD 2015b, 2015c, 2018a, 2018b). Alternative measures of homelessness in the Atlanta metropolitan area present a different picture, including unchanged rates of homelessness among some populations[1] that are 20 times higher than the Atlanta counts reported to HUD (Atlanta Youth Count 2015; Giarratano 2019).

Atlanta, like San Francisco, represents municipalities with a supportive housing policy, but it diverges from San Francisco on a few key characteristics of interest (Atlanta's population is majority Black, and Georgia as a state has not expanded Medicaid). As mentioned, in Atlanta the Continuum of Care, homeless policy governing system, became integrated into municipal government and homeless policy processes. Atlanta also adopted a municipal supportive housing policy as a result of institutional restructuring.

The Atlanta metropolitan area is comprised of 29 counties and the City of Atlanta (Metro Atlanta Chamber 2020). The Continuum of Care for the Atlanta metropolitan area used to be a combined Continuum of Care for three municipal jurisdictions within the larger Atlanta metropolitan area: Fulton County, DeKalb County, and the City of Atlanta. This arrangement was referred to as the "trijurisdictional" Continuum of Care. Atlanta's reform occurred when the Continuum of Care for the two counties and the City of Atlanta restructured, moving from the trijurisdictional arrangement to separate city and county Continuums of Care. The restructuring was prefaced by an investment in homelessness and chronic homelessness prevention and services by the City of Atlanta. Since then, the City of Atlanta has adopted a supportive housing policy and made the choice to oversee the new City of Atlanta Continuum of Care, integrating these policy processes. This chapter focuses on policy development and implementation for the City of Atlanta, including when Atlanta was a part of the trijurisdictional arrangement and afterward. However, as will be discussed, Atlanta's approach to chronic homelessness is directly influenced by its relationships with these overlapping municipal jurisdictions, including on-going barriers to supportive housing policy implementation.

Since the restructuring, Atlanta has made strides toward not only addressing supportive housing and reductions in rates of homelessness but also directly addressing criminalization responses to homelessness and the cyclical relationship between chronic homelessness and incarceration. Nationally, more than 20% of incarcerated individuals with severe mental illness are homeless in the months before their incarceration (Ware and Dennis 2013). In 2017, Atlanta established a Pre-Arrest Diversion pilot project to reduce quality-of-life (QOL) arrests, by diverting any arrests for QOL reasons (e.g., sleeping outside, eating outside, urinating in public) out of jail and into social services (the primary group affected by QOL arrests are people experiencing chronic homelessness; Macias 2017; Pre-Arrest Diversion Design Team 2017; Torres and Garland 2018).

Despite these important policy changes, Atlanta still suffers from se-rious barriers to policy implementation resulting from the histories of race and segregation, entrenched elite preferences, and limited state involve-ment. A strong, separate policy effort attempts to mobilize police services to move groups of persons experiencing chronic homelessness to other jurisdictions or away from desirable areas based on the preferences of or-ganized economic elites. Atlanta also faces significant funding challenges related to the history of Atlanta's Continuum of Care, limited governmental funding, and a reliance on nongovernmental actors as both providers and funders. As a result, the state and economic elite policy initiatives remain separate and constrain decision-making and policy implementation, while the institutional arrangements of Atlanta as a metropolitan area have direct, negative effects on all policy efforts and any policy coordination overall. In summary, the limited coordination between policy interests governing homeless policy reduces the implementation of publicly funded policy alternatives for Atlanta and increases the policy alternatives for pri-vately pursued reactionary policies.

HOW DID ATLANTA ADOPT A SUPPORTIVE HOUSING POLICY? SHIFTING INTERGOVERNMENTAL RELATIONS AND POLICY CAPACITY

Atlanta's movement to a municipal-level supportive housing policy occurred with the intersection of policy capacity and institutional restructuring. Unlike San Francisco (see Chapter 5, this volume), Atlanta began building policy capacity around homelessness specifically, instead of as a tangential social service or health area, which presented opportunities to focus on homelessness, as did HIV/AIDs and behavioral health in San Francisco. Once Atlanta established sufficient policy capacity in terms of funding, expertise, and awareness of homelessness as a municipal priority, the trijurisdictional Continuum of Care of the City of Atlanta, Fulton County, and DeKalb county separated in 2013 in an attempt to receive more federal dollars as independent entities rather than as a singular organization. The separation of the three trijurisdictional Continuums occurred three years after direct investment by the city of Atlanta in homeless policy. During this restructuring, governing members of the City of Atlanta realized they had the opportunity to either house the Continuum of Care as a governmental entity or keep it as a decentralized, nongovernmental entity as Continuums of Care have historically been organized. The choice to merge the Continuum of Care and municipal homeless policy efforts coalesced around local and national salience in supportive housing, urging Atlanta to adopt a supportive housing policy at the same time that the city had to define the local government's role in homeless policy.

Developing Policy Capacity

Atlanta began building policy capacity to address homelessness at the turn of the 21st century with the election of Mayor Shirley Franklin. The previous mayor, Bill Campbell, initially emphasized housing in the 1990s. The effort, however, ended in failure when it turned out that the programming was not only not successful but rife with corruption and direct interference from Mayor Campbell (Georgia Public Policy Foundation 1997; Sherman 2000). The election of Mayor Franklin helped increase tangible interest and efforts to address homelessness and chronic homelessness in Atlanta.

Mayor Franklin's efforts regarding homelessness prioritized municipal and philanthropic investment, promoting community organizations' efforts to address and prevent chronic homelessness (Franklin 2002). The effect that this had on Atlanta's policy capacity around homelessness, as well as on policy mobilization, was substantial. The Franklin administration's initiatives effectively developed Atlanta's current structure of community-based organizations that work together to manage homelessness in the metropolitan area.

Mayor Franklin initiated and leveraged partnership through the United Way of Metropolitan Atlanta to review current practices used to address homelessness in Atlanta (Deloitte Consulting 2003; Gateway Center's Commitment 2019; Tatum 2013). This review ultimately culminated in the

recommendation to create the Regional Authority on Homelessness to promote coordination across decentralized bodies of community-based organizations (Deloitte Consulting 2003, 1).

> "We found a huge number of people living in shelters for more than a year ... our
> [previous] Mayor Franklin was approached by the faith-based community, she
> asked the United Way to come up with a strategic plan because they work with
> corporations [to coordinate funding]."[2]

The Authority was eventually incorporated by the United Way (now the
Regional Commission on Homelessness), which now acts as a de facto and
parallel governing body for metropolitan-area homelessness planning and
service delivery, assisting with coordination across Continuum of Care
and metropolitan area jurisdictions (Gateway Center's Commitment 2019;
Tatum 2013; United Way Atlanta 2017). Thus, the Franklin administration's
efforts initiated movement toward a coordinated systems approach to
managing homelessness in Atlanta.

Although institutional efforts were primarily very decentralized, the
Franklin administration made strides toward formalizing municipal tax
structures as funding mechanisms to reduce homelessness by developing
Homelessness Opportunity Bonds through a rental car tax (although now
defunct; Atlanta Development Authority 2008, 8, 2009). The majority of
interviewees also emphasized that Mayor Franklin's work affected political
interests by successfully coordinating alliances across stakeholder groups
to prioritize homelessness as an issue of interest among both elected
officials and bureaucrats in Atlanta for the eight years she was in office
(Vogelsang-Coombs 2007, 222).

By the time Mayor Kasim Reed was elected in 2010, Atlanta had a
restructured and expanded network of nongovernmental organizations,
or community-based organizations, focused explicitly on addressing
homelessness.

> Mayor Reed saw homelessness was an issue, he was very active with influential
> people throughout the country ... he didn't just talk to people here, he reached
> out, that's why we got the Bloomberg grant, [it] funded other projects too, the
> 311 system, that was part of it, that really helped guide us to looking at it, as
> to how it [homelessness] can be fixed, we have this Bloomberg grant, let's get
> experts who know what to do.[3]

The expansion of the community-based organization space had the
dual effect of also creating a new base of organizations with an explicit

interest in homelessness. Community-based organizations were interested in homelessness by virtue of their existence and mission, as well as the fact that the expansion of nongovernmental actors had a vested interest in their own organizational success and commitment as employers. As a result, the community-based organization space became an increasingly active voice in homelessness policy and programming in Atlanta (Holland 2009). This activity almost certainly increased salience of the issue, acting as policy feedback to promote homelessness as a persistent political issue in Atlanta.

Following Mayor Franklin's work, Mayor Reed continued prioritizing chronic homelessness as a political issue in Atlanta. In 2011, Mayor Reed specifically sought out philanthropic financial assistance to address chronic homelessness in Atlanta and to further build policy capacity, attend to the city's financial limitations in dealing with chronic homelessness itself, and work to coordinate across the decentralized policy space (City of Atlanta 2011; Mayor's Innovation Delivery Team Atlanta Georgia 2014).

Mayor Reed began prioritizing solutions to chronic homelessness by enlisting consultation and financial support through a Bloomberg Philanthropies grant (City of Atlanta 2011; S. Jacobs and Torres 2013; Saporta 2011). The aim of the grant was to initiate coordination between Atlanta's municipal government and community organizations to address and reduce chronic homelessness and veteran chronic homelessness (City of Atlanta 2011; Mayor's Innovation Delivery Team Atlanta Georgia 2014; K. Reed 2014; Saporta 2011). This effort resulted in a significant growth in policy capacity, training over 100 providers in evidence-based supportive housing and vulnerability prioritization practices (S. Jacobs and Torres 2013; Mayor's Innovation Delivery Team Atlanta Georgia 2014). The investigation into and focus on chronic homelessness and systems coordination in Atlanta also led to a discussion about the governing structures. The Bloomberg Philanthropies funded Innovations project ultimately proposed a change to the Continuum of Care structure, generating momentum for reform and laying the groundwork for a greater municipal role (Pendered 2013). The proposed governing structure in 2013 included creating a separate governing council composed of local government and other stakeholders, which would direct policy and set priorities separate from but in coordination with the nongovernmental implementation bodies (City of Atlanta Innovation Delivery Team 2014; Governing Council of Continuum of Care 2017).

By 2013, when the Continuum of Care was actively restructuring, Atlanta had a larger policy space working directly on chronic homelessness and homelessness overall (Governing Council of Continuum of Care 2017). The policy space had expanded in terms of funding opportunities; efforts to recentralize or coordinate existing policy structures and programming; expansion of policy capacity via expertise based in community-based organizations and nongovernmental organizations dedicated to addressing different types of homelessness in Atlanta; and an overall growing political mobilization around the issue that had persisted since Mayor Franklin's election in 2000. The result of this continued mobilization and expanded policy capacity regarding homelessness and chronic homelessness in Atlanta was increased salience and attention to homelessness by municipal government and nongovernmental actors.

Continuum of Care Restructuring and Shifting Intergovernmental Relations

Following a decade of increasing levels of salience, political mobilization, and policy capacity around homelessness in Atlanta, opportunities for structural realignment began to appear. As mentioned, examination into Atlanta's homeless policy and programming by Mayor Reed led to an examination of the existing Continuum of Care structures (City of Atlanta 2011). This inquiry called for a greater role by municipal government in Continuum of Care governance to respond to needs for effective policy and program coordination across sectors (Governing Council of Continuum of Care 2017).

The opportunity for restructuring, however, did not become attainable until the trijurisdiction Continuums of Care began having discussions about their own funding and structural organization (Sheperd 2013).

> Well, [a nonprofit was] created by the city about three years ago [to be the Continuum of Care governing entity], but it was created in the midst of the breakup of a prior Continuum of Care which was a tri-jurisdictional Continuum of Care, which was Atlanta and two of our counties, so now all three municipal counties operate their own municipal Continuum of Cares, so. . . prior to that, it was a much different governance structure, the city was always supportive, but the city operated in a different way, so for the last three or four years, the city has been very supportive of the Continuum of Care and helped to establish it.[4]

The development of a formal role for the Atlanta municipal government in homelessness policy governance as a result of growing mobilization and policy capacity culminated in a structural realignment of the Continuum of Care. The trijurisdictional Continuum of Care broke up so the City of Atlanta would have its own Continuum of Care (City of Atlanta Continuum of Care 2015, 9). This decision forced municipal actors to choose between a direct municipal role or continued decentralization. The years of increasing interest by municipal actors in homelessness policy and programming, paired with increasing centralization across multiple spheres, allowed Atlanta to step into a direct municipal role when the opportunity arose. Overall, increased salience, substantial growth in homeless policy capacity, and movement toward centralization paired with structural realignment by intergovernmental partnerships allowed Atlanta to establish a formal municipal role in homeless policy.

All of the interviewees who were familiar with Atlanta's homeless policy discussed the restructuring of the Continuum of Care as a critical factor in municipal policy development, both in terms of establishing a formal role for the city of Atlanta as well as subsequently developing and establishing Atlanta's current supportive housing policy approach (Partners for Home 2017). The previous Continuum of Care (the trijurisdictional Continuum of Care) decided to restructure as a result of a shared funding stream. The trijurisdictional Continuum of Care ultimately decided shared federal funding mechanisms across the three municipal jurisdictions resulted in lower amounts of federal funding, compared to each independent jurisdiction applying for and receiving its own separate amount of federal funding (City of Atlanta Continuum of Care 2015; Partners for Home 2017). As mentioned, when discussions about Continuum of Care restructuring began in 2013, Atlanta had already heavily invested in homelessness policy and programming (Pendered 2013). The trijurisdictional restructuring decision, too, followed just two years after Mayor Reed had proposed a plan to formalize Atlanta's role in Continuum of Care governance (City of Atlanta 2011).

The restructuring ultimately aligned Continuum of Care governance with Atlanta's interest in and movement toward centralizing by locating an independent Continuum of Care in the City of Atlanta's jurisdiction, as opposed to the previous shared model. Locating an independent Continuum of Care within the City of Atlanta itself came with inherent questions about which authority would operate the Continuum of Care. Initial discussion prior to the 2013 decision suggested that the Continuum of Care would be overseen by an independent nonprofit.[5]

However, the change that ultimately occurred designated the Continuum of Care as a governmental entity, or a part of Atlanta's municipal bureaucracy, as opposed to a completely decentralized, nongovernmental entity (City of Atlanta Continuum of Care 2015, 152; Partners for Home 2017; Pendered 2013). This decision was made based on existing interest in coordinating homelessness policy in Atlanta, as a result of the growth in policy capacity and expertise to evaluate and improve homelessness systems, policy, and programming in the metro area (Governing Council of Continuum of Care 2017; Partners for Home 2017). Shifting authority to the City of Atlanta, as a result of the restructuring, inherently opened an opportunity for Atlanta to establish a municipal level policy on homelessness and chronic homelessness.

> 2013 is when they [Tri-j Continuum of Care] broke up. I don't know when the conversations actually started, but it was 2013 when the City of Atlanta formed Partners [new Continuum of Care governing organization]. So that would have been when Mayor Reed was already mayor. And, shortly [after] . . . they carried out, in 2013, as part of Unsheltered No More, a homeless registry, the first comprehensive registry to count people and count unsheltered, that is the pilot for coordinated entry.[6]

After establishing a formal municipal role, the movement toward a supportive housing policy happened relatively quickly. Since 2015, Continuum of Cares have been required by the federal government to apply a Housing First approach (Goodloe 2015). This federal policy change aligned with many of the policy goals and initiatives established by Mayor Reed, all following in a trauma-informed, supportive housing approach to specifically address Atlanta's high rate of chronic homelessness (Governing Council of Continuum of Care 2017; Partners for Home 2017). Ultimately, Atlanta's strong foundation in policy capacity, the establishment of a specific governance role for the City of Atlanta following institutional restructuring, as well as national policy change governing the Continuum of Cares themselves all acted together to push Atlanta toward a municipal level supportive housing policy in 2017 (Governing Council of Continuum of Care 2017; Torres and Garland 2017).

Without the previous development in municipal level policy capacity, including funding and expertise, Atlanta may not have felt prepared as a municipality to step into a formal governance role when the Continuum of Care restructuring occurred. Similarly, without the Continuum of Care restructuring, it is not clear that Atlanta would have taken steps to formalize a municipal role and ultimately a municipal level supportive housing policy, due to the strong history of decentralization both in Atlanta and in homeless policy and programming nationally. Most likely, we can assume that Atlanta may have eventually formalized a more indirect municipal role, as was originally laid out in Mayor Reed's plan for a municipal seat in the governing board overseeing the Continuum of Care, but not seating the Continuum of Care within Atlanta's city government itself. This case, as in San Francisco, posits the necessity of both policy capacity and institutional, intergovernmental arrangements as critical factors in promoting, or disincentivizing, municipal level homelessness policies. Policy mobilization to spur policy capacity and institutional realignment helped Atlanta move away from a fully decentralized (delegated to nongovernmental actors) model of homeless policy governance, providing the Continuum of Care with the authority and capacity to carry out its tasks to end homelessness and chronic homelessness.

JURISDICTIONAL BOUNDARIES AND THE HISTORIES OF RACE AND RACISM

Now that we understand why Atlanta developed a formal municipal role in homeless policy governance and a municipal supportive housing policy, we must examine how the policies work on the ground and if they work toward their intended goals. Despite Atlanta's success in policy design and policy capacity, one of the city's primary challenges to policy implementation, decision-making, and any service coordination is the existing municipal jurisdictional boundaries. These jurisdictional boundaries exist as a product of the histories of race and racism in the segregated South (Bayor 1988; Bullard, Johnson, and Torres 1999; Bullard, Johnson, and Torres 2000; Jackson 2009; Kruse 2005).

The interviews and archival analyses all showed that coordinating policy and service distribution across multiple, overlapping municipal jurisdictions results in: collective action problems, questions of authority and responsibility, coordination challenges, and deliberate gatekeeping mechanisms. As a result of the challenges posed by the jurisdictional boundaries, supportive housing policy implementation stagnated. Local supportive housing policies and other evidence-based solutions for chronic homelessness do not currently work to their intended ends and face the risk of not succeeding in the future. Municipal fragmentation in Atlanta compounds coordination challenges across policy sectors, contributing to fewer viable policy opportunities for publicly funded supportive housing efforts and increasing the alternatives to private actors by promoting the interests of segregated jurisdictions.

Why Does Atlanta Have Multiple Overlapping Jurisdictional Boundaries?

Atlanta exists within five separate incorporated counties—Fulton, DeKalb, Gwinnett, Cobb, and Clayton. This arrangement is not typical. Most cities exist within one county or sometimes two overlapping counties. Atlanta's arrangement is a product of direct segregation efforts to establish areas outside of the city that were (and are) primarily inhabited by white, wealthy elites, separated from and outside of the Black, poor, metropolitan downtown city (Bayor 1988; Kruse 2005). Atlanta's white flight is not unusual. Cities across the United States, including Detroit, Cleveland, Queens, and New Orleans, experienced great migrations of white, wealthy elites out of metropolitan areas during the mid-late 20th century as a result of increased racial animus by whites during the civil rights movement and white responses to direct efforts to reduce segregation. In effect, whites responded to growing economic mobility by Black Americans and increased desegregation efforts, with further segregationist efforts including escaping to the suburbs where they could insulate themselves through Federal Housing Administration redlining and racially discriminatory private business practices (Biles 2011; Frey 1979; Kruse 2005, 169).

Atlanta substantially grew and established the perimeters of its protected, white suburbs out of reach of Black America in the 1960 and 1970s (Bayor 1988; Bullard, Johnson, and Torres 1999; Kruse 2005). With this came the establishment of new governments (school boards) and separate governance and decision-making structures, all run by this new, separate group of wealthy whites (Frey 1979; Mickey 2015). The effect of expanding existing and creating new, separate governing entities that overlapped jurisdictionally with the City of Atlanta was done not only to perpetuate racial animus and segregation in the American South but to also engender further fragmentation of political decision-making and inherent challenges for governance of collective problems within the Atlanta metropolitan area (Bullard, Johnson, and Torres 2000). Today, this fragmented decision-making protects white, wealthy elite interests at the expense of lower-income, poor, and racial/ethnic minority groups or often socially constructed "deviant" outgroups, constraining coordination across policy interests—in particular intergovernmental relations—and inhibiting successful supportive housing policy implementation.

Collective Action Problems and Policy Coordination

The first challenge observed as a product of multiple, overlapping municipal jurisdictions in supportive housing policy implementation is an inherent collective action problem. The collective action problem arises because, although the City of Atlanta is a separate entity from the other municipal jurisdictions, three of the municipal jurisdictions serve the same, or strongly overlapping, populations. These jurisdictions are the City of Atlanta, Fulton County, and DeKalb County. This is because persons experiencing homelessness, and chronic homelessness in particular, may be mobile or migratory around metropolitan areas for a variety of reasons (Gray et al. 2011; Metraux, Treglia, and O'Toole 2016; R. D. Parker and Dykema 2013). These reasons include forced mobilization by municipal authorities to dissuade individuals from entering certain areas or clustering (Mcnamara, Crawford, and Burns 2013); mobilization caused as an after-effect of incarceration; the need to access services that are located in different municipal areas (e.g., city vs. county administrative processes required to obtain social services); among others (Gray et al. 2011). As a result of this mobilization, the closely overlapping jurisdictions within the larger metropolitan areas serve very similar or overlapping groups requiring/seeking services.

When working to address one collective issue, or a problem that simultaneously affects all overlapping jurisdictions, buy-in or some type of participation is required by all the areas to sufficiently address the problem and resolve the collective issue. This is particularly true in the case of chronic homelessness, which requires (and now is required by federal regulatory bodies) implementation of coordinated entry and assessment, along with an integrated and coordinated Homelessness Management Information System (HMIS; U.S. Department of Housing and Urban Development 2017a, 2020). These systems work to effectively identify and coordinate the flow of information across organizations to address clients' needs, identify clients with the highest needs to prioritize service access based on risk, and follow clients throughout the system to make sure those who are seeking help are able to receive aid and do not fall outside of the system (U.S. Department of Housing and Urban Development 2017a, 2020). Therefore, participation and buy-in from all jurisdictions within the metropolitan area is required to implement effective programming that can successfully execute supportive housing protocol and place individuals into supportive housing as well as connect them with other services.

A clear example of the collective action problems supportive housing policy implementation faces is the use of the HMIS across jurisdictions. Stakeholders mentioned that some individuals who have been in existing permanent supportive housing units for extended periods of time are stable and ready to transition out of these units, into other supportive but less intensive environments. This transition would then free up more supportive housing units for currently chronically homeless individuals. However, the lack of coordination across the jurisdictions has resulted in a fragmented HMIS network, where providers are unable to track unit availability, to help clients access services through the system.

> [Chronically homeless] people sit on the queue for over a year sometimes, and if no one has made contact with them in 90 days, they are bumped off the queue. That doesn't really make sense, and they are using it off of our [Atlanta Continuum of Care] HMIS, but not everyone uses that, so that person could have been touched by an agency but maybe that person didn't get into the system because that agency didn't use HMIS.[7]
> They will have like five beds over here, and seven beds from another county, [but they] can only fill beds for people living in certain county. It's weird how they decide.[8]

As it currently stands, the historic separation of the multiple jurisdictions within Atlanta's metro area acts as a barrier to collective action to employ evidence-based practice to address chronic homelessness. All interviewees stated that not all jurisdictions participate in homelessness programming and implementation, and, if they do, not all participate to the same degree. For example, Fulton was reported as typically less participatory or more absent from most decision-making and programming meetings.

Fulton County is the jurisdiction with the most overlap with the City of Atlanta. Further, Fulton County is the primary arbiter of public health services in the Atlanta metropolitan area, following traditional city/county arrangements of public health service delivery (Fulton County 2020). Lack of participation by Fulton County acts as a direct barrier to policy decision-making and implementation, as Fulton is not only a jurisdiction governing a core portion of the primary population but also a service provider. Therefore, limited participation by Fulton effectively constrains access to resources and governance structures necessary to implement supportive housing policy and homelessness services in the metropolitan area for the shared, targeted population.

> Now a lot of the difficulty is we have two Continuum of Cares [Atlanta and DeKalb] that are very active and participatory, and [homeless services] providers whether they like them are not are in communication with them, but then you have Fulton County that is in and out at best.[9]

This constrained coordination across governments reduces policy success and opportunities for evidence-based municipal policy efforts.

Overall, lack of participation, or comparably less participation, by any of the individual jurisdictions constrains action and effective governance on the part of the other jurisdictions due to the overlapping target population and the policy goals requiring coordination across systems to monitor service access and client needs. Multiple overlapping jurisdictions serving the same client population need to all buy in to decision-making and implementation or the system may not successfully deliver policies and track client needs.

Questions of Authority, Responsibility, and Gatekeeping

Beyond the inherent collective action problem, Atlanta's multiple jurisdictions also create questions of authority and responsibility that follow from or may perpetuate collective action problems. Interviewees frequently discussed challenges in determining which jurisdiction is responsible for which homeless population and how the reorganization of the Continuum of Care exacerbated some of these issues. Specifically, the reorganization moved from a singular system into a system that still serves an overlapping population and therefore requires coordination but is governed through three separate entities. In this way, the restructuring may have had a double effect: allowing the City of Atlanta to formally establish a municipal level policy, formal governing role for the city and through it expanded policy capacity, yet fracturing a system already facing jurisdictional challenges. Overlapping jurisdictions interacting with questions about authority remain at the crux of policy coordination challenges constraining municipal supportive housing policy opportunities.

The interviews highlighted a critical way questions of designated authority or responsibility for a shared target population primarily affect policy implementation. The effect is delineating boundaries of responsibility within each jurisdiction, where the lines dividing jurisdictions become gray zones of service gaps as well as create reduced visibility for individuals experiencing homelessness and chronic homelessness. These service gap zones, or zones where individuals experiencing homelessness effectively lose visibility or where homelessness becomes less salient, may also be used as a deliberate gatekeeping mechanisms to shift visible homelessness into less desirable areas. Deliberate gatekeeping via jurisdictional boundaries promotes elite policy interests while reducing policy success for evidence-based municipal Continuum of Care efforts. Deliberate gatekeeping is discussed more in the next section.

The question of authority or responsibility pertaining to service gaps works in two ways. One regards presumptively nondeliberate service gaps. Nondeliberate service gaps are a result of the jurisdictional boundaries, where services levels are inherently lower at the boundaries between jurisdictions compared to the center. As mentioned, there are many different reasons why individuals experiencing chronic homelessness may end up on the fringe of jurisdictional boundaries. The result, however, is that without an effective, coordinated approach across jurisdictional boundaries, individuals living on the boundaries of the jurisdictions receive fewer services and are often harder to track. In addition to structural service density, individuals living on the boundaries may also face service gaps due to the second type of mechanism behind service gaps.

The second way relates to deliberate service gaps, where different jurisdictions may or may not be responsible, or perceive responsibility, for different tasks in implementing supportive housing or take an overall coordinated approach to addressing chronic homelessness. The effect of deliberate service gaps on individuals living on the boundaries is a lack of certainty regarding which municipal jurisdiction is responsible for that population.

> The homeless congregate in the boundaries, e.g. North Cobb people congregate in this boundary between North Cobb and Cherokee . . . both sides want people to go on one side or the other, or across ends of a parking lot. Policing stays away from the edge. You can tell, you drive through the city and you can see that. You can see there will be a bulk of homeless people, those people probably aren't being served if they aren't in the city of Atlanta, agencies congregate in city of Atlanta, a lot of them [homeless] are on the boundaries.[10]

Often, the lack of certainty, according to interviewees, results in inaction. Inaction compounds the lack of service access and results in ineffective, or constrained, policy implementation specifically for individuals experiencing chronic homelessness who are living in the boundaries between municipal jurisdictions. This subsequently perpetuates the collective action problem facing supportive housing policy implementation by constraining policy implementation resulting from limited coordination across policy interests.

Finally, the deliberate service gaps may also be a product of or directly related to deliberate gatekeeping mechanisms. Deliberate gatekeeping mechanisms are discussed more completely in the context of the local political economy in the Atlanta metropolitan area. However, the ability of these gatekeeping mechanisms to exist is directly related to the municipal jurisdictions. All of the interviewees discussed the use of some deliberate gatekeeping mechanisms by jurisdictions in the context of keeping persons experiencing chronic homelessness out of less desirable areas. Specifically, interviewees said that individuals who live between jurisdictions have less visibility, which may be more desirable to some stakeholders or jurisdictions, overall aligning with negative social constructions of homelessness often pursued by economic elites (see Chapter 2, this volume). In effect, these results question the relationship between deliberate service gaps between jurisdictions and elite stakeholder preferences. The next section evaluates how municipal fragmentation exacerbates policy coordination challenges across policy interests, interacting with elite preferences to increase available policy alternatives for private actors while constraining policy alternatives for municipal efforts.

ECONOMIC ELITES AND POLICING—PARTICIPATORY EQUITY

Atlanta's municipal supportive housing policy, as well as specific efforts to decriminalize homelessness and chronic homelessness, have not yet translated into successful policy implementation. In particular, Atlanta's new municipal homelessness decriminalization efforts have not ceased a primary challenge supportive housing and decriminalization policy implementation wrestles with: the relationship between policing and homelessness in Atlanta's metropolitan area.

The relationship between policing and homelessness in Atlanta cannot be separated from the relationship between wealth and policing. Similar to the situation in San Francisco, this research finds that the processes surrounding informal policing of persons experiencing homelessness (outside Atlanta's decriminalization initiatives) are a product of the police responding to or carrying out preferences of wealthy stakeholders in the metropolitan area. Regarding policy implementation, the interviews and archival analyses all demonstrated that policing efforts as directed by wealthy stakeholders result in (1) direct barriers to service access and homelessness programming roll-out and (2) growing participatory inequity in the Atlanta political economy. The challenges posed by policing, and institutional arrangements prioritizing elite preferences over at-risk or policy-targeted populations, stymied supportive housing policy implementation and intended policy goals.

The relationship between policing and homelessness in Atlanta currently occur on two axes. The first is efforts to decriminalize QOL crimes, which persons experiencing chronic homelessness are typically cited for. In Atlanta specifically, one 1 of every 10 chronically homeless individuals was housed in jail on any given night (Fulton County 2012, 13). QOL crimes include behaviors resulting from behavioral health disorders (sleeping in public, eating in public, etc.) or all crimes that are a direct result of being homeless and are not in and of themselves a product of criminal behavior or intentions (Macias 2017). Atlanta started a pilot program that redirects persons who have been charged with a QOL crime out of jail and into social services to address the causes of the QOL crimes in the first place (Macias 2017). Atlanta also eliminated bail for QOL crimes, so individuals experiencing chronic homelessness (or poverty) are not held in jail simply because they are unable to pay bail for a misdemeanor (Torres and Garland 2018). Finally, the police are often the first point of contact for individuals experiencing homelessness. In response, the Atlanta Police Department developed a Homelessness Outreach Proactive Engagement (HOPE) team as a means of training police officers in crisis intervention and in delineating between crisis behavior and criminal behavior and to connect individuals experiencing chronic homelessness and other types of homelessness with social services.

Despite these notable efforts, stakeholders in Atlanta consistently reported a different relationship between policing and homelessness. This secondary axis, or relationship, is one that is responsive to the interests of wealthy or influential members of the public or constituencies within Atlanta and acts as a means of addressing the visibility of homelessness—or behaviors associated with homelessness—as opposed to connecting individuals with services or addressing the causes of chronic homelessness. Interviewees emphasized that although new policing efforts seek to shift toward a compassionate approach, policy conflict and institutional constraints hinder change. As discussed, Atlanta faces limited resources for sufficiently addressing the causes of homelessness. High levels of influence from economic elites exacerbate the effects of resource constraints on policy implementation by redirecting evidence-based policing goals to relocate individuals experiencing homelessness out of visible areas. Overall, current policing reforms have not been able to overcome the substantial implementation challenges borne out of the reactive relationship between policing and homelessness.

Barriers to Service Access and Programming

The reactive relationship between policing and homelessness in Atlanta mirrors that of San Francisco. Police officers react to calls or complaints about homelessness from actors, notably wealthy or influential actors, and in response enact protocol to respond to those complaints, which typically encompasses responding to behaviors associated with homelessness.

Responding to behaviors associated with homelessness is often antithetical to evidence-based harm-reduction approaches that focus on providing services that are required for implementing supportive housing or Housing First. These responses most often include moving homeless encampments—persons and possessions—out of desirable areas into less desirable areas of the city.

Elite requests through policing between Atlanta and San Francisco are different in one important way. What is notably different in Atlanta compared to San Francisco is that local economic elites as a stakeholder group in Atlanta appear to be comprised of corporate interests as opposed to wealthy individuals or independent citizens. This composition is similar to local elites in Shreveport, Louisiana (see Chapter 7). Yet, the outcomes and processes involved in police responses to homelessness in San Francisco and Atlanta are very similar.

Just as in San Francisco, when organized elites in Atlanta interact with police, the process generates or acts as an additional, independent policy mechanism—both decision-making and implementation—separate from other policy mechanisms developed and intended to address homelessness through the municipal Continuum of Care and local supportive housing policy. In the separate policy process, organized elites' preferences in Atlanta guide direct responses to homelessness, addressing homeless visibility or homeless behaviors as opposed to the causes of homelessness. As discussed, this policy goal directly contradicts and conflicts with the goals of supportive housing policy, while also working through independent decision-making mechanisms and implementation processes. The separation and conflict between these policy goals and processes generate inherent barriers to supportive housing policy implementation. Organized elites with high levels of political capital access police, and receive quick responses, through informal, nonpluralistic policy mechanisms. Individuals experiencing chronic homelessness are often pushed out of areas where they are able to access supportive social and medical services, typically perpetuating homelessness as opposed to addressing the causes of homelessness.

All interviewees discussed three main ways elite actors promote alternative policing policy processes and responses: (1) external corporate interests (movies and sporting events), (2) municipal downtown development organizations (housing and other), and (3) the history of wealth and racial segregation in Atlanta. In these ways, organized elites' preferences are often bolstered over other interests, including racial/ethnic minorities and persons at risk of or experiencing homelessness, through institutional constraints such as municipal fragmentation, limiting opportunities for other actors to participate or share their preferences. In the end, organized elites have more available policy opportunities, and municipal supportive housing policy efforts face reduced, viable policy alternatives as a result of successful elite interventions conflicting with or counteracting supportive housing policy processes.

External organized corporate entertainment interests are a growing presence in Atlanta. Corporate entertainment interests are different from Atlanta's downtown development stakeholders. What delineates these interests from downtown development is they are often external actors who do not reside in Atlanta but have a vested economic interest in Atlanta for an acute period of time. From the interviews, the two most commonly cited types of organized corporate elites are movie productions and national sporting events. While the introduction of these groups into Atlanta's economy is arguably positive for many reasons, these prominent stakeholders represent one mechanism for catalyzing isolated elite policy efforts, conflicting with supportive housing policy processes. These elite policy processes are informal and opaque and have no enforceable accountability mechanisms. "Police are running the streets, when things happen, when a convention happens, when Super Bowl . . . like we just did, we know, as we did from the Olympics, the community doesn't want to show its negative side, so they sweep the problems [homelessness] away."[11]

The majority of interviewees were not aware of the mechanisms by which police responses were activated, for example, whether the City of Atlanta calls police on behalf of these external interests or these groups alert the police of their preferences. Regardless, interviewees all stated that immediately prior to the arrival of external, corporate interests—notably film crews, the Olympics, and the Super Bowl (Gustafson 2013; Smothers 1996; Stokes 2019)—individuals experiencing chronic homelessness or visible homelessness (e.g., living and sleeping on downtown streets individually or in encampments) are removed from areas (or areas that will be utilized by external elites), as are their belongings. "Officers use [QOL ordinances] to sweep them [homeless] off the streets, almost all of them [ordinances] were put in place in order to sweep the streets for the Olympics."[12] The areas that are typically affected are downtown areas—areas where homelessness services and programming are primarily located.

Many interviewees stated explicitly that their clients are not returned to the downtown, or their original locations, after these corporate elites leave Atlanta. As a result, providers cannot locate their clients, and clients are not able to access homelessness services and programming and are many times completely disconnected from the systems of care overall. Some interviewees stated that, after the Olympics, many persons experiencing homelessness were never located and are still missing from the local supportive housing systems.

> No one is saying anything, there are lots of horror stories of the '96 Olympics, bussing people out of town to an abandoned military base out of town, we think they are doing it again [before the 2019 Superbowl], but very quietly, we keep seeing police everywhere doing quiet sweeps, police come into camps [homeless encampments] and finger print people.[13]

This is a clear example where organized, corporate elite preferences were promoted not only over the success of municipal supportive housing policy efforts but to the detriment and livelihood of persons who are chronically homeless. These findings align with previous research on the interactions between policing and chronic homelessness in municipalities across the United States (Mcnamara, Crawford, and Burns 2013).

Downtown municipal development interests are the second group of organized elites interviewees cited as a primary catalyst for reactive police responses to chronic homelessness. Downtown municipal development refers to the growth of new, generally more costly infrastructure, typically owned by large corporations or entities, in the city of Atlanta itself. This includes new residential property, as well expansions for other uses developed by existing downtown entities such as Georgia State University. These interests differ from the former as they are entities that reside in Atlanta and have long-term developmental interests and relationships in the city. I refer to them as "entrenched" economic elites.

Downtown development, too, is growing in Atlanta and is also arguably good for Atlanta's economic growth in many ways (Kahn 2019). However, the introduction of new, wealthy political actors into Atlanta's downtown political economy through informal policy mechanisms reshapes Atlanta's political economy. Similar to external elites, entrenched elites leverage informal political participation networks through policing, constraining input by other constituencies as well as the targeted population. These reactive, fast-acting policy mechanisms occurring in narrow civic networks also place direct barriers to supportive housing policy goals and implementation. Interviewees cited efforts by both new residential properties and Georgia State to remove individuals experiencing homelessness from or near their properties, to the same effects as the external elites: displacing individuals into areas with low access to homelessness services and programming and limiting the ability to reach clients and coordinate access to supportive housing and other services to ameliorate homelessness.

Finally, the history of wealth and segregation in Atlanta exacerbates elite influence through informal policy channels on homelessness policy and programing in Atlanta. Atlanta, as discussed in the previous section, has a long history of racial and economic segregation, by and through which the municipality's overlapping jurisdictions developed (Kruse 2005). Interviewees stated that when these organized elites—both external and entrenched—enact policing procedures to remove individuals experiencing chronic homelessness, such individuals are typically moved to specific parts of the Atlanta metropolitan area. These areas are historically segregated, low-income, and low-service areas. Interviewees stated that this is generally in south Atlanta, past highways 75 and 80.

> So, we don't actually move them [people experiencing homelessness] around, if you drive under 75/80 right now, there are encampments there. Somebody calls and complains, if the right person sees it, we have to go, we let them [homeless] know you have 24 hours to move your stuff, in 24 hours we come and get rid of things, it's really whoever calls and complains. It's a really reactive profession [policing], so the proactive part of that is really nonexistent.[14]

Moving individuals experiencing chronic homelessness to racially and economically segregated and overall disadvantaged areas of Atlanta stagnates supportive housing policy implementation by moving individuals further away from outreach and service efforts. These actions also inhibit individuals experiencing homelessness from returning to serviceable areas themselves, by sequestering them off from other services including transit, food systems, and medical care. The history of and contemporary structural arrangements of wealth and race in Atlanta, in conjunction with the elite policy mechanisms, protect elite preferences while insulating at-risk population's preferences from the larger political economy and simultaneously restricting supportive housing policy implementation.

> [The public transit system] is segregated by race and by class, people who use public transport are more at-risk of homelessness than people who don't. There is direct opposition on extending the subway system, into different more suburban neighborhoods, in places where they were concerned about bringing more poverty in [to their neighborhoods] . . . being a behavioral health provider, it's a huge issue a lot of patients are trying to use public transit and they can't get to their appointments on time.[15]

In these ways, organized elites' preferences are often bolstered over the interests of persons at risk of or experiencing homelessness, through institutional constraints such as municipal fragmentation, limiting opportunities for other actors to participate in policy processes. Overall, organized elites have more policy opportunities and municipal supportive housing policy efforts face reduced viable policy alternatives as a result of successful elite interventions targeting behaviors associated with homelessness through reactive policing, conflicting with or counteracting supportive housing policy processes.

Growing Inequity in Atlanta Political Economy

As discussed, Atlanta's political economy has always been inequitable due to the history of slavery and segregation in the South (R. D. Bullard, Johnson, and Torres 1999; R. D. Bullard, Johnson, and Torres 2000; Kruse 2005; R. Mickey 2015). This section highlights the role of the history of inequity and segregation in Atlanta, compounded by a new, changing political economy in downtown Atlanta. Extending from the previous section, this research finds that increasing income inequality is exacerbating inequity in political participation by structurally limiting homeless, racial minorities, and low-income groups' access to wealthy or gentrifying areas in the Atlanta metropolitan area. Engendering inequality through structural arrangements—neighborhood or jurisdictional segregation—in Atlanta may perpetuate threats to successful supportive housing policy implementation and further fragment the existing and conflicting policy approaches between local government and economic elites.

As a product of historic segregation, the city of Atlanta is surrounded by wealthy, primarily white suburbs (Kruse 2005). In contrast to San Francisco, all interviewees in Atlanta, overwhelmingly, insisted that there is no direct opposition by any entity to supportive housing policy or homelessness services and programming generally. What interviewees did state, however, is the history of segregation in the Atlanta metropolitan area has provoked strong feelings of protectionism among wealthy suburban areas. As a result, instead of direct opposition to homelessness or supportive housing development as seen in San Francisco, Atlanta experiences opposition to development that would further economic integration or improve mobility for residents experiencing homelessness and low-income residents into wealthy neighborhoods. These trends have been demonstrated in urban politics literature, where white enclaves are more protectionist and often have stricter zoning rules as mechanisms to protect intraneighborhood homogeneity (Bates and Santerre 1994; Trounstine 2020). This typically comes in the form of strong opposition to subway expansion or expansion of the transit systems in general (Rankin et al. 2015).

> Expansion of MARTA discussions have been ongoing. This is the bus service and train . . . it's really limited, bus service is really slow, it takes a long time, Atlanta is very segregated economically, those [segregated/wealthy] populations voted down expanding MARTA, lots of really racist arguments were made against expanding MARTA . . . it's a really frustrating thing because it could help Atlanta become a lot more integrated economically.[16]

As a result of this historic segregation and protectionism, or NIMBYism ("not in my backyard) among suburban elites, most low-income individuals and individuals experiencing homelessness and chronic homelessness reside in downtown Atlanta (City of Atlanta Continuum of Care 2015; Holt and Lo 2008; Pearce et al. 2016). What this research finds are increasing concerns among stakeholders about growing inequality in downtown Atlanta, which threatens to push low-income, at-risk, and homeless or chronically homeless individuals out of downtown, further out of Atlanta jurisdictions, creating greater housing insecurity. Interviewees working in homeless policy and programming in Atlanta stated that they anticipate rates of homelessness in Atlanta to rise due to the changing economy in downtown Atlanta in the coming years.

The compounding effects of historic segregation and increasing gentrification in Atlanta may have an effect similar to that in San Francisco. The result may be an exodus of marginalized communities out of metro Atlanta, and out of the political economy. These two parallel forces work to increase inequity in Atlanta's political economy by further limiting marginalized communities' ability to participate in policy debates by removing them from the metropolitan area. This trend is not uncommon and was used very intentionally in major metropolitan areas during the mid-20th century as a way to decrease political participation by less desirable out-group members (Bridges 1999; Galster 2012; Sugrue 2014; Trounstine 2008). Political debates thus become inherently inequitable or biased toward the dominant group if another group is ousted or has constrained access to political debates. A restructuring of the political economy toward a more homogenous group of wealthy individuals may result in less support for municipal supportive housing policy by constraining buy-in from groups that would benefit from municipal supportive housing efforts, increasing policy alternatives for private actors.

Summary

The existence of these two separate policy processes in decision-making and implementation—elite and municipal—with fundamentally separate policy goals leads to further stagnation of efforts to address homelessness by crowding the policy space with multiple competing policies and actors that all directly contradict each other's efforts. These policy processes, similar to those in San Francisco, structurally engender inequality. The mechanism by which these processes occur—request by one individual (or single entity) through informal channels for action regarding chronic homelessness—allows no time for input or political participation from other entities or actors. It simultaneously creates a siloed and one-sided policy response to chronic homelessness that also substantially affects other actors' goals and abilities.

BARRIERS TO POLICY IMPLEMENTATION: BRINGING THE STATE BACK IN AND IMPROVING MUNICIPAL ACCOUNTABILITY

Atlanta's municipal supportive housing policy and targeted efforts to de-criminalize homelessness and chronic homelessness have not yet translated into successful implementation. A primary challenge restricting policy implementation in Atlanta is a lack of funding and challenges pertaining to the *utilization* of existing funding. The funding challenges occur in two main domains: (1) limited state participation and (2) the local government's use of funds and local funding initiatives.

The State of Georgia is relatively absent from Atlanta's choices related to policies addressing chronic homelessness. As of 2017, Georgia was entirely absent on the front of legislation or funding directly targeting homelessness. This limited participation by the State of Georgia exacerbates existing challenges in the city of Atlanta. Atlanta relies on little to no municipal resources for homelessness programming. The majority of funding for homeless programming in Atlanta comes from philanthropy (City of Atlanta Continuum of Care 2015; Hobson 2019). In addition, Atlanta's history of corruption and limited transparency around the use of federal dollars for supportive housing and other efforts in the City of Atlanta Continuum of Care (Deere 2018, 2019) further strain limited resource capacity for solutions to chronic homelessness. As a result, much of the federal funding leveraged to fill the gaps in municipal and state funding has come under scrutiny due to questionable uses or a limited return on investment (Deere 2018). The challenges posed by funding constraints at the state and local level create barriers to supportive housing policy implementation and efficacy. This section argues that solutions to these challenges may come in the form of improved coordination between the state, local elites, and the municipal Continuum of Care, to align policy goals, reduce participatory inequity, and establish systems of accountability.

Bringing the State Back In

All interviewees stated that Georgia, as a state, is relatively absent from municipal level homeless policy concerns. One interviewee noted that Atlanta is a system that has so few municipal and state level resources that it relies very heavily on private funds.

> The corporations of Atlanta . . . Georgia isn't known for its state funding or county or city government for this [homelessness] issue. So, we raised lots of private money with the agreement that we wouldn't take away from the HUD money. Mostly private money here.[17]

The reliance on private donations allows Atlanta to be more innovative, yet the tradeoff is a lack of sustainability and consistency to effectively achieve policy goals over a long period of time. Interviewees emphasized that more resources from the state would be greatly appreciated by municipal actors.

As of 2017, Georgia had no state-level policies addressing homelessness or chronic homelessness.[18] Georgia has also not expanded Medicaid and does not have any existing Medicaid waivers to be used as funding or pilot funding for supportive services or issues tangential to homelessness and chronic homelessness such as low-income risk pools (Centers for Medicare and Medicaid Services 2019). In San Francisco and Shreveport, interviewees highlighted Medicaid funding as a major asset for supportive housing policy development, despite implementation challenges (see Chapters 5 and 7). In Atlanta, the majority of interviewees described the lack of state funding overall as a barrier to supportive housing policy development and implementation. Municipal-level actors and providers also outlined Medicaid expansion as a missed opportunity for additional state-level funding to facilitate local supportive housing policy efforts.

> We haven't expanded Medicaid, so paying for the services is really challenging. We are thinking through a sustainability plan for 550 units of PSH . . . we are developing right now. . . . Oh, and beyond the Medicaid, sustainability in terms

of other public resources to homelessness, we have no dedicated state or local dollars for investments in homelessness.[19]

Despite these drawbacks, there was a high level of policy mobilization among municipal-level actors unique to Atlanta compared to San Francisco and Shreveport (see Chapters 5 and 7). This policy mobilization is specific engagement by local-level actors, both political and bureaucratic, to seek out and advocate for state-level resources to assist in homelessness and supportive housing policy and programming. Interviewees stated that their efforts to seek state-level resources were motivated by a dearth of municipal governmental funding and historically limited federal funds for the Atlanta Continuums of Care, which is discussed more in the next section. Interviewees felt that some state-level resources could be made available that would help support their efforts given absent or constrained municipal and federal funding.

> The state Department of Community Affairs funds some programs through passthrough CDBG grants, behavioral health and disabilities, provider vouchers for people with mental health. . . . There has been now more a concerted effort [from the state] to partner with Partners for Home [new Atlanta Continuum of Care] . . . they fund physicians to fund PATH [Projects for Assistance in Transition from Homelessness] outreach teams.[20]

These municipally driven efforts to seek state funding have proven fruitful so far. As mentioned, local actors have been able to leverage additional support for behavioral health services. Local actors stated that the relationships with state-level bureaucrats in these agencies are growing, and they are hopeful that these relationships will continue to increase state investment in local homeless policy initiatives to fill funding gaps. Local actors in Atlanta may have been more willing to seek out state-level funding compared to San Francisco and Shreveport as a result of the highly constrained funding environment at the municipal and federal levels.

The history of policy conservatism in Georgia (Lassiter 2006; R. Mickey 2015) makes future participation in welfare or social service funding unlikely. However, in recent years, state-level representation and public opinion has been changing. Aside from potential swings in public ideology and representation, policy diffusion from other conservative states regarding Medicaid expansion through waivers may increase the likelihood of Georgia taking an interest in Medicaid expansion alternatives. Atlanta's Continuum of Care has also taken an active role in lobbying Georgia for the benefits of Medicaid expansion (Partners for Home 2017).

The changing political environment, paired with an increasing relation-ship between municipal and state actors, may ultimately move the policies toward greater alignment and may help Atlanta's municipal level sup-portive housing efforts work better to their intended ends (Lillvis and Greer 2016), creating more policy opportunities for municipal supportive housing policy efforts.

Municipal Accountability and Funding

Two distinct barriers to supportive housing policy result from (1) Atlanta's *available* funding for homelessness programming and (2) Atlanta's *use* of funding for homelessness programming. The first refers to two is-sues: Atlanta's history of limited federal Continuum of Care funding and a history of inadequate or absent municipal level funding for homelessness programming and policy (e.g., taxation, bonds, etc.). The second refers spe-cifically to Atlanta's murky relationship with federal funding as a product of the muted transparency around spending federal funding and a history of corruption.

When the Continuum of Care funding streams were formalized by the federal government in 1995, local communities were required to iden-tify a "Continuum of Care" in order to submit a single application for federal funding (U.S. Department of Housing and Urban Development 2012). Before the passage of the McKinney Vento Act in 1987, most communities already had some type of organization among community groups overseeing homelessness programming, and therefore the formal transition to a Continuum of Care was less challenging. Atlanta, however, was late to the game. Although there is limited documentation and litera-ture on this topic, interviewees underscored that Atlanta's slow decision to establish a Continuum of Care substantially reduced the metropolitan area's baseline amount of funding, as the initial amount was formally tied to establishing a Continuum of Care. The downstream effects of this choice constrain Atlanta's resources for homelessness programming, requiring the municipality to look elsewhere for funding sources.

From what I understand, when the Continuum of Care funds first came out in the '80s, Atlanta didn't go after the money initially, they were slow to apply, that made a big difference . . . just from day one essentially, if you didn't apply in the beginning, you had a lower dollar amount at a later date, we started out at a disadvantage, you can only increase in bonus dollars . . . Continuum of Cares can only grow in small increments every year.[21]

Despite the reality of limited federal funding, Atlanta has a history of limited municipal governmental efforts to levy local funds to address homelessness. There has been opposition to taxation, in particular, as a funding source.[22] Other municipal funding in Atlanta has been limited to public-private partnerships, with the majority of municipal funding coming from philanthropic or corporate investments (Atlanta Development Authority 2009; Torres and Garland 2017). The United Way has been one of the largest sources of funding, acting as both a partner providing match funding for municipal investments as well as a source of staffing for municipal bureaucracy dedicated to homelessness programming and the Continuum of Care itself.

> [With the Continuum of Care restructuring] . . . until the dollars were available for that [the United Way] funded it and staffed it until the resources were coming in in a more sustainable way, [the United Way] funded it for a year or two, providing staffing still now, but not to the same degree.[23]

This limited municipal governmental funding may be surprising, given the constrained federal funding opportunities. However, the growth of the submerged state as a primary funder in this hampered arrangement is less surprising (Weir and Schirmer 2018, 382). All interviewees emphasized that the reliance on nongovernmental sources of funding presents barriers to supportive housing implementation, because funding sources are not sustainable. Therefore, much programming goes unfunded or is not implemented, especially in the way of building more supportive and/or affordable housing units.

In this narrow funding environment, there are two additional barriers shaping municipal supportive housing policy implementation. These two constraints may be related to the history of a limited governmental role or the major role that private or nongovernmental actors play as funders and contractors in Atlanta's homeless policy and programming. These additional barriers are a history of corruption and reduced transparency around homeless policy governance and funding allocations. In a strongly delegated state, even with a newly established role for municipal government incentivizing greater centralization and oversight, delegated private actors have their own interests that may contradict policy goals. These interests may be easier to conceal in a delegated state with limited transparency and oversight (Hackett 2017; Mettler 2016; Weir and Schirmer 2018).

The majority of interviewees, unprompted, cited corruption and or misuse of appropriated public or (private funds for public use) by public officials as a major challenge to homeless and supportive housing programming and policy in the City of Atlanta. In Atlanta, corruption in housing and homelessness policy and programming, specifically, ruled the city in the 1990s (Deere, Trubey, and Klepal 2018; Jarvie 2006). Since then, rumors of corruption in the Franklin administration and Reed administration, and new charges of corruption among the current Bottoms administration, are an undercurrent continually tying elected officials to staffing bribery schemes and unauthorized uses of municipal funds (Cardinale 2014; Deere 2019). Most recently, the Bottoms administration had 2017 Continuum of Care funding withdrawn as a result of misuse of federal funds (Deere 2018).

An environment of limited governmental funding, and a strong reliance on nongovernmental actors not only as service providers but as funders themselves, engenders a state of limited transparency and oversight of public investments. Continued reliance on private dollars, as a result of a strong delegated state and a history of limited governmental investment, presents barriers to supportive housing policy implementation. Despite Atlanta's work establishing both municipal level supportive housing policy and decriminalization legislation, the lack of transparency and accountability create threats that must be addressed for policies to function effectively. Without sufficient oversight mechanisms, decentralization reduces successful municipal supportive housing policy alternatives and promotes policy alternatives for private actors as a result of concealed, conflicting interests.

SUMMARY

Atlanta is a case where the Continuum of Care has become integrated into municipal government and homeless policy processes. Atlanta, too, also came to have a municipal supportive housing policy by way of institutional restructuring. Atlanta's reform occurred when the Continuum of Care restructured, moving from a trijurisdictional arrangement to separate city and county Continuum of Cares. The restructuring was prefaced by an investment in homelessness and chronic homelessness prevention and services in Atlanta by the city itself. Since then, the city has adopted a supportive housing policy and made the choice to oversee the new city of Atlanta Continuum of Care, therefore officially integrating these policy processes and homeless policy governance as a municipal endeavor.

Despite these policy changes, Atlanta still suffers from substantial constraints on policy implementation resulting from the histories of race and segregation, entrenched elite preferences, and limited state involvement. There still exists a strong, separate policy effort mobilizing police services to coordinate an indirect and informal policy space of moving groups of persons experiencing homelessness to other jurisdictions or away from desirable areas based on the preferences of organized economic elites. Finally, Atlanta faces significant funding challenges related to the history of Atlanta's Continuum of Care, limited state policy coordination and governmental funding, and a reliance on nongovernmental actors as both providers and funders. The state and economic elite policy initiatives remain separate and constrain decision-making and policy implementation as a result, while the institutional arrangements of Atlanta as a metropolitan area have direct negative effects on municipal supportive housing and decriminalization policy efforts and policy coordination overall. Ultimately, fragmentation across policy sectors governing homeless policy responses reduces the implementation of publicly funded policy alternatives for Atlanta and increases the policy alternatives for privately pursued, reactionary policing policies.

CHAPTER 7

The Delegated State

Shreveport and Challenges of Authority and Capacity

WHAT'S HAPPENING IN SHREVEPORT?

This chapter focuses on Shreveport, LA, a case with little to no municipal involvement, where responsibility to address homelessness and chronic homelessness in the city lies with nonprofit, nongovernmental organizations. San
Francisco and Atlanta both have an integrated homeless governance system
that is a part of their respective municipal governments and coordinates
with other relevant municipal offices to promote evidence-based, supportive
housing efforts. Why has Shreveport not been able to achieve this, and what
are the implications of this delegated governance system for local homeless
policy efforts? This chapter will focus on explaining why, as compared to San
Francisco and Atlanta, Shreveport experiences little to no municipal governmental involvement in homelessness policy and programming or supportive
housing policy and (1) outlines the barriers to municipal governmental involvement and (2) the influences of the barriers resulting from the lack of
a municipal role on the current supportive housing efforts put forth by the
Continuum of Care, the local homeless policy governance system.

Introducing Shreveport

Shreveport is a medium-sized city in northwest Louisiana with about
200,000 residents (Data USA 2020c). The poverty rate in Shreveport (in

Ungoverned and Out of Sight. Charley E. Willison, Oxford University Press (2021). © Oxford University Press.
DOI: 10.1093/oso/9780197548325.003.0007

2020) is more than twice the national average at 25.7% of the municipal population. Once a hub for the oil industry, Shreveport experienced a high rate of job loss in the 1980s and has not been able to recover, despite new growth in the natural gas industry (Brendler and Jones 2000). The majority of Shreveport's population identifies as Black (56.4%); 37.5% identify as white, with Hispanic or Latino and Asian residents making up less than 3% of the population (Data USA 2020c). According to the U.S. Department of Housing and Urban Development, there were 390 persons experiencing homelessness in Shreveport in 2015 (U.S. Department of Housing and Urban Development [HUD] 2015f). In 2018, there were 375 (HUD 2018f).

Unlike San Francisco and Atlanta, Shreveport serves as the representative case for municipalities without a municipal government level supportive housing policy. Thirty percent of the cities in the national data set (see Chapter 4, this volume) without a supportive housing policy matched the same criteria (variables) as Shreveport. Shreveport is a case where the Continuum of Care (CoC) and the local government remain very separate in homeless policy decision-making and in practice, especially when compared to the integration seen in Atlanta and San Francisco. This separation, in policy design and practice, was the most prominent theme among interviewees. The Continuum of Care in Shreveport has strong policy capacity and, despite of limited municipal involvement, has made great strides in reducing homelessness in Shreveport. Yet in the face of this success, the lack of local government involvement presents continuous barriers to supportive housing policy design and implementation for the Continuum of Care by limiting their authority and the resources available to the Continuum of Care to pursue and execute homeless policy and solutions to chronic homelessness.

Beyond the separation of municipal government and the Continuum of Care, Shreveport also experiences a strong influence from economic elites that engenders further barriers to supportive housing policy similar to San Francisco and Atlanta. Organized economic elites act as informal policy mechanisms outside of local government decision-making and Continuum of Care activity to unofficially govern the activity of individuals experiencing chronic homelessness through elite requests for police department action to manage homelessness. Most of this police activity is punitive and contradicts Continuum of Care policy and evidence-based homelessness reduction programs (Poremski, Whitley, and Latimer 2014; Robinson 2019; University of California Berkeley School of Law Human Rights Center 2017). As discussed previously, although police departments are a part of local government infrastructure, this action by elites is classified as a separate policy process because the policy mechanisms function in a different manner compared to all other types of local government policymaking (legislation, ballot initiatives, and regulation). The Continuum of Care in Shreveport has taken steps to curb such police activity, but these efforts are not formal policy and have not been widely effective due to the limited participatory ability of the Continuum of Care as nongovernmental actors.

Finally, the State of Louisiana also remains separate from local homeless policy decision-making, as is the case in San Francisco and Atlanta. Shreveport sees more direct state-level policies that offer to provide tangential support for homelessness policy and programming, especially chronic homelessness. Yet, severe resource constraints facing Louisiana overall negatively affect many state-level efforts, perpetuating misalignment between state and local initiatives and act as further barriers to local supportive housing policy efforts.

Overall, Shreveport presents a case of a strong delegated state with few incentives for municipal governmental participation in local homeless policy. An absence of incentives for municipal involvement are exacerbated by participatory inequity in local governmental decision-making; racial tensions and racism; and limited state involvement that fails in implementation.

FORMALIZING THE ROLE OF THE DELEGATED STATE

Shreveport is a case of nearly full delegation of homelessness policy and programming to nongovernmental actors. The City of Shreveport, based on archival results and interviews, does not participate in homeless policy implementation and has very limited involvement in decision-making. The Continuum of Care, HOPE for the Homeless, acts as the primary governing entity for homeless policy and programming in Shreveport and the regional area[1] (City of Shreveport Louisiana 2016). The designation of the Continuum of Care as the main governing entity means that the Continuum of Care designs policy priorities regarding responses to homelessness, decides how federal Continuum of Care dollars (3 to 4 million dollars a year; U.S. Department of Housing and Urban Development 2018c) will be used, and works with other local nonprofit organizations that are a part of or work with the Continuum of Care to implement homeless policies such as coordinated entry, permanent supportive housing units, etc.

The primary role of the City of Shreveport, from 2002[2] onward has been to act as a pass-through organization to distribute federal funding for the Continuum of Care. This federal funding includes Community Development Block Grant funds, Housing Opportunities for Persons with

AIDS, and Continuum of Care Emergency Solutions Grants (ESG) (City of Shreveport Louisiana 2016).

> The city itself does very little . . . [the] Department of Community Development has passthrough money through ESG funds, so we can access that funding, but the Department of Community Development doesn't have a clear understanding of how that funding needs to be used.[3]

Beyond allocating federal funding, there have been fewer than ten instances between 2002 and 2019 of city council or mayoral deliberations or decisions pertaining to homelessness in the city of Shreveport (City of Shreveport Louisiana 2019).

The first instance was a long deliberation over nearly two years from 2014 through 2015 debating whether or not to allow the Continuum of Care to use public land to build a new homeless shelter. Interviewees emphasized that this was one of the few times that the city was involved in homeless policy decision-making. Interviewees also cited that the Continuum of Care received strong pushback when trying to gain permission to build the new shelter despite serious capacity constraints at the original shelter location. Ultimately, in 2014, the city council agreed to authorize the mayor to execute a cooperative agreement for the Continuum of Care, HOPE for the Homeless, to utilize a public lot in Shreveport to construct the new shelter (City of Shreveport Louisiana 2014).

The second major instance was in 2012 when the city council agreed to reallocate 87,000 dollars from the Farmers Market fund to the Continuum of Care for homeless services programming (City of Shreveport Louisiana 2016). Other instances include a few deliberations over constructing low income housing developments, the development of a 10-year plan for homelessness in 2005 (which there is limited archival documentation at the municipal level on whether or not this was completed and what actions may have stemmed from this), and two debates over declaring November as Homelessness Awareness Month (Everson 2014).

The near-complete absence of policy debates regarding homelessness at the city level validates interviewees statements that the City of Shreveport is, in practice, essentially uninvolved in local homeless policy. The city is more involved in tangential policy spaces including affordable housing through the Shreveport Housing Authority, regarding distribution of federal affordable housing funding, and parish-level Medicaid administration via Medicaid expansion enrollment efforts. Yet, overall, the results demonstrate that Shreveport stands as a direct comparison to the policy models in Atlanta and San Francisco where there has been deliberate and purposeful integration of municipal government and the Continuum of Care to direct, oversee, and implement local homeless policy and programming.

This research was not able to find a record of a statutory designation of authority for homeless policy and programming to the Continuum of Care by the City of Shreveport or Bossier Parish. In addition, this research was also unable to find records of the historical development of Shreveport's Continuum of Care. Based on the extant literature, Shreveport's informal delegation of authority to the Continuum of Care would align with federal homeless policy and the history of decentralization and neoliberalism in U.S. homeless policy overall (Jones 2015). Prior to the McKinney–Vento Act in 1987, most municipalities did not formally address homelessness (Grob 1994). Culturally, homelessness was thought to be the responsibility of families or community organizations. The development of the Continuum of Care's was argued to be a natural extension of the existing community or nongovernmental structures that had been historically responding to homelessness (Grob 1994; Jones 2015; Cronley, 2010). Therefore, in many municipalities across the United States, cities' roles in addressing homelessness may not come out as a question, due to the institutionalization of the Continuum of Cares as the main arbiters of homeless programming and the policy histories of limited role for municipalities in many parts of the United States (Jarpe, Mosley, and Smith 2018).

In summary, this research finds that across the past 20 years to the present Shreveport has retained very separate municipal government and Continuum of Care in homeless policy processes. The ways that this separation plays out in practice, regarding political decision-making and policy implementation, has notable implications for homeless policy governance. These implications shape who decides, what policy options are available, and how homeless policies are implemented and overseen. The bifurcation also ultimately influences the success of various homeless policy goals, such as effectively introducing and implementing coordinated entry, supportive housing or Housing First.

THE VOLUNTARY WELFARE STATE: MECHANISMS OF DELEGATION

The results of the interviews and archival analyses reiterate that Shreveport is a case of complete delegation of homelessness policy and programming to nongovernmental actors. As previously discussed, this delegation may not be entirely surprising given the history of homelessness policy in the United States and the alignment with conservative ideals of welfare state governance (Soss, Fording, and Schram 2011; U.S. Department of Housing and Urban Development 2009). What this section discusses, following from Shreveport's history of delegated authority to nongovernmental actors, is how this delegation affects policymaking in decision-making and implementation. This section also evaluates Shreveport as a case of the implications of complete policy delegation for homelessness policy outcomes. To date, most of the research on delegated authority to nongovernmental actors in different welfare policy spaces has focused on identifying and measuring degrees of delegation, which actors comprise the delegated state, and the processes leading up to the choice to delegate away from government. This section also adds to the literature on the delegated or submerged state by providing empirical evidence of the *mechanisms* of the delegated state at work in active policy processes.

The most striking result from the case analyses was that nongovernmental or Continuum of Care interviewees stressed their absence from most local policy decision-making. Interviewees expressed that this absence was not desired on their part as stakeholders in homelessness policy but a reality in Shreveport due to the overall absence of any local government authority in homelessness policy decision-making or programming. Beyond a general absence, interviewees also emphasized their difficulty accomplishing tasks directly related to homelessness policy or programming as a result of limited to no access to local governmental processes or decision-making. In effect, constrained political participation and reduced political leverage across Continuum of Care actors introduced barriers to homelessness policy and supportive housing implementation in Shreveport or reducing policy alternatives for publicly funded efforts.

The majority of interviewees cited local government's general absence in homelessness governance and programming. The absence, interviewees stated and archival analysis reflects, comes in the form of: staffing or monetary resources, bureaucratic expertise and formal opportunities for political participation. The City of Shreveport provides no municipal-level monetary resources for homelessness policy or programming (City of Shreveport Louisiana 2016). Staffing is explicitly directed to the Continuum of Care. Bureaucratic expertise or policy capacity for homeless programming is also delegated to the Continuum of Care (HOPE Connections 2019b; Shreveport Downtown Development Authority [DDA] 2019).

In practice, the Continuum of Care does attempt to coordinate with the city regarding Community Development Block Grant funding and for housing vouchers through the Community Development Department. However, the Continuum of Care does not directly receive Community

Development Block Grant funding. Further, the Continuum of Care relies heavily on private donations to fill in gaps in federal support and due to the lack of local or state funding. "We can't do it without the federal funding, but sometimes there is a disconnect with boots on the ground. . . . One of our largest funders is the Community Foundation [a private funding entity]."[4]

Regarding bureaucratic policy capacity and staffing, the Continuum of Care remains relatively separate from the city regarding meeting attendance and homelessness policy governance. The majority of decision makers and attendees at Continuum of Care monthly meetings who provide essential policy capacity to support federal designated goals come from nongovernmental actors in the local area (HOPE Connections 2019b).

Considering formal opportunities for political participation, the majority of interviewees stated that they as Continuum of Care member organizations or stakeholders had never been invited to a municipal governmental meeting. Interviewees also emphasized that the bulk of instances where local government does reach out to the Continuum of Care is not about homeless policy or planning but in response to elite complaints, primarily organized private actors, about the presence of individuals experiencing homelessness in downtown business districts.

> The only time I've ever been called to a meeting with the city council to talk about issues of homelessness, I was like, sweet, maybe the city will start doing something, awesome, and they called us in and they said that they had complaints about people pooping in the doorway of the Courthouse, and I was like that's all you want to talk about, and so we were like we could really use money for a low-barrier shelter, and nothing ever came of that.[5]

This prioritization of very different interests reiterates the separation of the Continuum of Care and city government, where the Continuum of Care prioritizes evidence-based homeless reduction initiatives and the city's limited participation prioritizes policy discussions driven by economic elites focused on addressing undesirable behaviors associated with homelessness and chronic homelessness.

Following from reduced opportunities to participate in political decision-making, most interviewees described participatory inequity for the Continuum of Care compared to municipal actors in policy spaces necessitating participation for the Continuum of Care to successfully carryout homeless programming. In effect, Continuum of Care actors have very limited opportunity to participate in municipal policy debates. Yet,

Continuum of Care actors require municipal resources and access to municipal decision-making to implement homeless policy and programming. Such municipal resources include debates on building permitting or zoning ordinances for construction of Continuum of Care space and affordable housing, local funding initiatives, and policing. Overall, the participatory challenges Continuum of Care actors face to enter municipal policy spaces present ongoing barriers to any homeless policy implementation, let alone supportive housing policy.

The most frequently cited example of participatory inequity interviewees discussed was the case of building the new Shreveport Continuum of Care shelter. Prior to 2015, Shreveport did not have a singular homeless shelter that had the ability to offer and coordinate food services, social services, and medical and housing needs (Brumble 2013; Durden 2015). The Continuum of Care at the time was working toward adopting a coordinated entry system for homelessness management (City of Shreveport Louisiana 2016). The Continuum of Care decided that to begin moving toward a coordinated entry approach it needed a shelter that provided a "one-stop shop" for individuals experiencing homelessness. This one-stop shop would allow individuals experiencing homelessness to register for social services, register with the Continuum of Care and begin receiving medical aid and other vital services without having to travel to multiple locations across the city. A centralized registration process would also allow the Continuum of Care to track clients and prioritize their needs based on federal vulnerability scales to implement coordinated entry and begin moving toward supportive housing or Housing First programs.

When the Continuum of Care began working through the permit approval process, they faced substantial pushback from city council members, the Community Development Department and the private Shreveport DDA. Overall the discussions from the interviews demonstrated that a lack of participation or a seat at the table in municipal policy debates inhibited the Continuum of Care's ability to lobby for their case to construct the shelter. The strong economic alliances between the private business community and city council further exacerbated existing participation disparities facing the Continuum of Care.

The original challenge the Continuum of Care encountered in this process regarded the location of the shelter. The Continuum of Care wanted to build the shelter downtown, to promote ease of access to services for individuals experiencing homelessness. Interviewees described that ultimately strong pushback from the DDA and limited input from the Continuum of Care resulted in the Continuum of Care changing their request for permitting downtown to different location.

I don't know if you're familiar with how Shreveport is. The city wanted to revitalize the downtown, but at the same time other people wanted a lot of homeless out of downtown—fund the day shelter that is like five miles away. It's always very political.[6]

The new location was over one mile away from downtown and proved difficult to access for low-income or homeless individuals facing transportation constraints. The shelter was built in 2015, after delays related to permitting and due to funding shortages (City of Shreveport Louisiana 2014, 2015). The political participation constraints facing the Continuum of Care directly conflicted with Continuum of Care policy goals to promote coordinated entry and federally mandated goals to provide coordinated entry and work toward Housing First by inhibiting policy implementation and creating new barriers related to transportation and access, ultimately serving the policy preferences of economic elites.

The second, most prominent theme interviewees cited as a constant policy barrier directly related to participatory inequity or limited Continuum of Care authority are police relations. Currently, under federal regulation, Continuum of Cares must be working to reduce criminalization of homelessness to continue to receive federal funding (Tars 2015). In practice, the absence of any municipal governmental role for the Continuum of Care makes this mandate not feasible. The majority of interviewees cited continual challenges between Shreveport and Bossier parish police officers regarding criminalization responses to homelessness, management of homelessness, and barriers to implementing Continuum of Care coordinated entry practices. Criminalization responses include police jailing or citing individuals for quality-of-life crimes or behaviors related to mental illness; management of homelessness including relocating individuals to less desirable or accessible areas; and coordinated entry barriers including attempts to work with police officers to redirect individuals experiencing homelessness to the Continuum of Care instead of jail or hospital emergency departments. Overall, interviewees described requests for police reform through primarily educational outreach but an absence of any firm policy.

So that has been a continual challenge and I'm sure it is elsewhere. We have tried to work with community police, we've done education with them, and we try, we have a program where they have community liaison officers, that individual really tries to integrate into a certain part of the city and learn who the individuals are who are homeless, as you know it becomes a revolving door because they don't want to arrest them because they have to house them and [there are] no options when they get released [from jail]. It is very difficult . . . but you get a new officer who tries to jump to that arrest versus looking at options that are available.[7]

Continuum of Care actors without municipal authority cannot require police officers to make any policy or practice changes regarding homelessness. Interviewees stated that the Continuum of Care continually offers trainings for officers on engagement practices, quality-of-life crimes, and responding to mental health crises or behaviors. Interviewees stated that while they have had luck with some individual officers, they face uncertainty regarding the police department as a whole and ongoing challenges in educating new recruits or transfers. The lack of any authority or greater political participatory equity places Continuum of Care policy in a voluntary state. Continuum of Care actors may be required to promote or work toward certain policies and practices, but in cases of primary policy delegation, participation from municipal actors who are vital to the implementation process remains voluntary.

The absence of any local government participation in homelessness policy, paired with severe constraints on political participation for Continuum of Care members, ends in the reality of a voluntary policy space. Complete delegation of homelessness governance translates into a policy space where regulations governing the Continuum of Care cannot be translated into practice as a direct result of the limited to no authority Continuum of Care actors have over any municipal services, or other private or nongovernmental actors, to coordinate policy implementation effectively. Continuum of Cares in this space can only ask and hope for buy-in from critical actors. In cases where actors governing housing resources, zoning, and building permitting, police activity and even county or parish level health insurance enrollment choose not to participate, homelessness policy and programming may fail or stagnate with serious consequences for persons experiencing homelessness and local economies (Willison 2017). Under complete decentralization, without any real Continuum of Care governing authority, homelessness policy and solutions to chronic homelessness under the delegated state remains voluntary, limiting public policy opportunities.

The voluntary status of the current delegated state of homeless policy in Shreveport and many municipalities across the United States assumes adequate levels of policy capacity and action by the local Continuum of Care. Shreveport is a case where the Continuum of Care is very strong and has been able to make strides in reducing homelessness due to their adoption of a coordinated entry model of service delivery (prioritizing the most vulnerable first; HOPE Connections 2019a). Even with this strong Continuum of Care model seen in Shreveport, as outlined in this chapter, the Continuum of Care faced very substantial challenges to implementing these policies, reducing punitive police responses to homelessness, and building more housing infrastructure. Other literature has demonstrated notable heterogeneity in Continuum of Care service capacity and gaps in service delivery nationally (Jarpe, Mosley, and Smith 2019). In municipalities with the same characteristics as Shreveport, where the municipality is not involved but the Continuum of Care does not have strong policy capacity, the effects of delegation and a limited municipal role may pose greater challenges to homeless policy implementation by further constraining policy alternatives. Further inhibiting the local homeless governance system will presumably have stronger implications for the health and well-being of individuals experiencing homelessness and chronic homelessness, and those at risk of homelessness.

POLICING, ECONOMIC ELITES, AND RACE

The previous section outlined Shreveport's history of delegation of homelessness governance to nongovernmental actors and the practical implications of this delegation to the functions of homelessness policy. This section will consider the role of elites in further fragmenting the decentralized policy space and exacerbating implementation challenges for the Continuum of Care. In Shreveport, organized elites function very similarly as in Atlanta and San Francisco. Wealthy elites and business owners make formal or informal complaints with police officers, who respond by reacting to homeless behaviors either through statutory functions or informal activities like removing persons experiencing chronic homelessness from desirable areas or business districts.

What is very different in Shreveport compared to San Francisco and Atlanta is that without a formal governing mechanism for the Continuum of Care through the local government, the Continuum of Care as stated has no authority or leverage over police activity and cannot review current practices or make any kind of acute or long-term reforms. The absence of formal Continuum of Care roles and constrained political participation for the Continuum of Care has led to a challenging relationship between police officers and the Continuum of Care. The entirely voluntary reform efforts on the part of the police department regarding policing and punitive responses to homelessness also developed from this institutional relationship. The police department, or municipal corrections, are not discussed as community partners in any of the Continuum of Care's recent annual action plans to HUD (City of Shreveport Louisiana 2016, 2017). Similarly, with little to no oversight of police activity and limited viable mechanisms for reform, Shreveport interviewees discussed issues of racism and/or bias against individuals with severe mental illness (SMI). Both of these issues have serious consequences for the treatment of individuals experiencing chronic homelessness, while also creating substantial barriers to implementing homelessness policy and programming and/or best practices including supportive housing and coordinated entry.

As previously mentioned, policing homelessness in Shreveport works through very similar mechanisms as in San Francisco and Atlanta. The primary mechanism interviewees discussed is wealthy elites and business owners (i.e., private actors), issuing complaints to police officers. Interviewees outlined that the complaints usually pertain to the presence of persons experiencing homelessness in the downtown district. Business owners are typically the most common complainers, because they have concerns that the presence of homelessness dissuades patrons from entering their businesses. Many people experiencing homelessness spend time downtown because of access to services and transportation. Organized business also issues complaints about homelessness in the downtown district. This refers to the DDA, which will both submits complaints to city council to encourage greater police responses to homelessness and direct requests to police officers to increase enforcement in the downtown core.

> [The] DDA is very vocal against homeless people in Shreveport, as far as taking away benches downtown so there's no place to sit, that was the City Council, the DDA had pressure on the Council to do that, you know you've hear about all of the weird anti-homeless city ordinances, you can't do whatever, I know our folks get harassed a decent amount.[8]

Interviewees stated such private actors, businesses and organized business, have a disproportionate influence on policy activity responding to homelessness related to the Continuum of Care's constrained authority and ability to participate in local government.

The second type of interactions police officers have with persons experiencing homelessness is through patrols. In the instance of patrolling, interviewees described police interaction being initiated as a result of behavioral health symptoms including substance use disorders and/or SMI. Patrolling may also initiate responses based on police judgment of misdemeanor infractions, which usually pertains to loitering. Interviewees emphasized that loitering citations are usually issued specifically to their homeless clients, who have nowhere else to go beyond outdoor, public locations. "A lot of repeat arrests. . . . It may be getting arrested for loitering, and if you're out on parole, then you get thrown back in jail, very minor like that, sleeping on a park bench."[9]

As touched upon previously, police officers respond to these complaints made by organized, private actors in a number of ways. The different responses have varied effects on individuals experiencing homelessness. Loitering is the most common citation interviewees highlighted that their clients experience as a result of police interaction. Many interviewees discussed the burden of these minor citations, where homeless clients typically end up with multiple loitering tickets because they have no other place to go, are waiting for social services, the bus, etc. and may be subsequently incarcerated for failing to pay the tickets as a result of income constraints.

> I can tell you what we experience with our patient population, if they got a transportation problem, if there is someone who has been incarcerated before, they have to pay a monthly fee they have to pay, then they will arrest them again. I wish I could give you the right terminology, if they are released early, but there is the monthly fee they have to pay, I don't know if it's the Parole Board, fifty, thirty bucks a month, if they can't pay that fee they get picked up again. I've seen that someone was supposed to be at clinic, but they've been re-arrested.[10]

After loitering, there are a number of police responses in Shreveport that vary in severity. As in San Francisco and Atlanta, police will remove individuals experiencing homelessness from downtown Shreveport to less desirable and accessible parts of the city in response to elite requests. Removing individuals from downtown reduces their access to services and public transportation. This removal requires individuals experiencing homelessness to travel further to receive services and/or for health and social service outreach teams to travel further to establish interactions. Even if outreach teams reach these individuals, accessing services remains challenging for individuals if they remain in these out-of-reach areas as it is harder for them to travel from the local to various service area locations. This removal also has the additional, unintended consequence of deterring some individuals from receiving services at all. Interviewees cited that some persons experiencing chronic homelessness become so disenchanted with police interactions that they retreat to other, highly inaccessible locations such as wooded areas, preferring to live off the grid than face consistent pushback against their attempts at accessing housing and medical services.

Beyond removal, individuals experiencing chronic homelessness may also be jailed for a variety of quality-of-life infractions, including sleeping in public, eating in public, urinating in public, etc. Jail creates even greater barriers for individuals experiencing homelessness and homelessness policy overall as a result of repeating cycles of incarceration and re-entry, where persons are disconnected from services upon re-entry and not appropriately reconnected with services or the Continuum of Care system after discharge from jail. The lack of appropriate re-entry service coordination often leads individuals to be re-incarcerated for failure to treat behavioral health symptoms or address homelessness (Ware and Dennis 2013). Interviewees emphasized that individuals experiencing homelessness and SMI are disproportionately incarcerated in Shreveport and Bossier (HOPE Connections 2003).

> Of course, people with mental illness, that is criminalization of mental health issues, ... but if we had hospitals like we needed, that would cut down a lot. There are a lot of people who cycle between jail and homelessness—it's about 60% of our clients, it may be higher, 60% at least—[we] see our clients in and out of jail all the time—especially at the behavioral health unit ... and it's nothing more than mental health—they get stabilized, get out and end up right back in [jail].[11]

Interviewees also discussed the same result for people of color, explicitly citing segregation and racism as influential factors. The wealth disparities that exist in Shreveport exacerbate this, where low-income individuals in Shreveport are disproportionately Black, and low-income and Black individuals face higher rates of homelessness (Data USA 2020c; U.S. Department of Housing and Urban Development 2018f).

The final type of interaction between police and people experiencing homelessness are shootings. San Francisco and Atlanta did not discuss police violence. The majority of interviewees in Shreveport discussed negative or inappropriate responses to persons experiencing homelessness by police, with a few discussing explicit, violent responses to persons experiencing chronic homelessness. Interviewees cited police shootings as a response to persons who are homeless and suffering from SMI. A commonly cited incident was a recent incident where a long-term client of the Shreveport Continuum of Care was shot in a casino after being released from jail. The client was schizophrenic and was not currently on appropriate medication after re-entry. When the police responded, the individual was not able to cooperate with orders as a result of his schizophrenia. Police officers perceived this to be a threat and shot and killed the client.

> "We had a client that had been in and out of our system for about a year, schizophrenic, had delusions, he was involved in criminal justice system. ... I guess

it's been about a year ago now, he was at a local casino, he was banned but they called the police, he was delusional, our client went for officer's gun, and he was shot and killed. We had . . . tried to have him involuntarily committed, about two weeks before, it's just, our system is so broken, when it comes to people with high mental health needs, it's sad that his life ended that way.[12]

Interviewees used this as an example of the lack of awareness and training among Shreveport police officers on appropriate responses to behavioral health crises. Interviewees outlined that a lack of initiative among police and the lack of authority for the Shreveport Continuum of Care[13] to institute any trainings or reforms as primary reasons for inappropriate or violent police interactions with persons experiencing homelessness and SMI.

These interactions between police and individuals experiencing homelessness, paired with the engagement constraints Continuum of Care actors face in coordinating with local police, present adverse consequences for chronically, homeless individuals as well as direct barriers to homeless policy implementation. Direct effects on individuals include barriers to accessing services resulting from removal from economic zones or incarceration, while also facing direct threats to mortality in the cases of shootings of persons suffering from SMI. The effects on individuals are directly related to the effects on homeless policy implementation. The Continuum of Care's limited authority as nongovernmental actors restricts their ability to review police interactions and initiate efforts to implement federal regulations aimed at reducing punitive policing responses to homelessness and promoting supportive housing. In Shreveport, complete decentralization of the Continuum of Care and thus their limited ability to restrict harmful police behavior aligned with private business interests restricts policy alternatives for the Continuum of Care and increases alternatives for organized elites through informal and formal mechanisms. In San Francisco and Atlanta, where homeless policy governance is centralized as a part of local government, police and the homeless services work together to create policies formalizing preventative measures integrating evidence-based approaches, even in the face of completing elite interests.

MEDICAID EXPANSION REALITIES AND IMPLEMENTATION CHALLENGES

Like San Francisco and unlike Atlanta, Shreveport is a case where the state of Louisiana policies exist and run parallel to the Continuum of Care policies.

What this means, is that Louisiana has policies in place that are related to or provide support for individuals suffering from SMI and/or homelessness; or resources and funding to support health services and behavioral health programming related to homelessness and SMI. These policies center around Medicaid expansion and alternative Medicaid waivers. These are not all of the policies that may be related to supportive housing policy and programming however, these are the two policies that stakeholder interviewees specifically identified and emphasized the influence of these policies on local level policy decision-making and implementation.

As discussed in San Francisco, Persons experiencing chronic homelessness have often been considered prime candidates to benefit from Medicaid expansion; many individuals are high-need and were previously ineligible for Medicaid as single adults (Dipietro, Artiga, and Gates 2014; Warfield, DiPietro, and Artiga 2016). Addressing chronic homelessness requires complex interventions that simultaneously manage behavioral health needs, including SMI and substance use disorders, with other medical needs and housing instability. Decades of research have shown that supportive housing—specifically Housing First, which provides housing without behavioral prerequisites to housing access such as sobriety—is the most successful intervention for ending chronic homelessness (Kertesz et al. 2016, 2115). Medicaid expansion not only could increase access to medical services, but because of the enhanced funding mechanism, could allow states to open up new pots of money to address other pressing needs such as homelessness.[14] As such, the focus of this section is the interaction between local homeless policy efforts in Shreveport (supportive housing and Housing First) targeting chronically homeless adults and Medicaid expansion in Louisiana.

The existence of these Medicaid policies is an important first step and one that offers alternative resources and funding opportunities for Continuums of Care and communities looking to address homelessness in Louisiana. However, even though the state-level policies target homeless populations and supportive medical services related to supportive housing policies, in practice the state-level policies have different goals and work through different mechanisms to design and implement policy compared to the Continuum of Care in Shreveport. For example, Medicaid policy is developed through regulatory mechanisms at the state level with federal oversight through the Centers for Medicare and Medicaid Services. Medicaid policy is implemented through local county (here, parish) public health offices. Medicaid goals are centered around behavioral health interventions and healthcare coverage. These mechanisms and goals are very different compared to Continuum of Care governance structures and policy goals. This divergence creates (1) administrative barriers and (2) funding constraints that effectively engender implementation challenges for Continuum of Care actors working toward supportive housing policy. These challenges are compounded in Shreveport, where the nongovernmental homeless governance system faces greater barriers to coordinating with other levels of government, local and state, by virtue of their decentralized authority and position. This further inhibits the Continuum of Care's ability to align Medicaid and homelessness policy goals and mechanisms and reduces policy opportunities for the Continuum of Care.

Without working to align policy goals and processes between state and local initiatives, supportive housing programming and policy in Shreveport will continue to face implementation challenges. This effect is compounded by an overall absent municipal government where state-level funding and programming could fill this gap. Simultaneously, misalignment of these intergovernmental policies may further disincentivize municipal level actors from becoming more engaged in homelessness policy and programming by offering limited rationale and no downward pressure for policy engagement in terms of resources, requirements, or oversight.

Administrative Burden

The policy space that the majority of interviewees cited as having the greatest influence on local homelessness policy and practice is Louisiana's Medicaid expansion. Most interviewees emphasized that Medicaid expansion, overall, was beneficial for the state and provided access to new resources for persons experiencing homelessness—in particular, chronic homelessness. The reality of these new resources, though, is not ease of access to resources that sufficiently support local homelessness policy efforts. Nearly half of interviewees described challenges stemming from Medicaid expansion administration that simultaneously improved access to resources and services while also engendering new policy implementation barriers and short-lived benefits for individuals. Archival documentation illustrated similar challenges related to Medicaid expansion implementation and homelessness. All in all, the evidence outlined challenges for supportive housing policy presented by Medicaid expansion as a product of state-level policy design that did not adjust or work with local level implementation practices and were not designed to adapt to inherent challenges posed by homelessness. Most of the design adaptation problems were associated with administrative features that (1) do not align with local-level needs or practices and (2) directly contradict or create implementation challenges for homelessness specifically.

Half of interviewees and all provider interviewees emphasized the challenges inherent to the discrepancies between local systems implementation and/or capacity and state-level Medicaid requirements for implementation. This administrative misalignment ends in administrative burdens on local entities attempting to manage Medicaid billing and services to fund homelessness policy and programming and provide clients access to services or billing challenges resulting from state-level administrative burdens that do not align with local implementation practices.

For example, the majority of the agencies that provide homelessness services and programming in Shreveport are small, nonprofit, and nongovernmental organizations. Interviewees detailed the challenges that these organizations face in working to bill Medicaid, due to the high administrative requirements to file and contest Medicaid reimbursements for different services. Further, many of these organizations face challenges related to sustaining Medicaid as a payer due to their inability to afford, as an organization, the infrastructure and resources to actually bill and manage Medicaid claims. This is exacerbated in certain types of claim circumstances. For example, interviewees outlined that case management services tend to be more challenging to bill for Medicaid compared to traditional medical services, often facing multiple claim rejections that require a higher administrative infrastructure to dispute the rejections.

> The [case management] billing has proven difficult, in fact the, LA put our some housing that used Medicaid case management as "match," two main agencies, our providers of that have had a very difficult time keeping it afloat. It's very expensive to do Medicaid billing, to get reimbursements, so your agency's too small, we almost have to have a third-party billing company to bill Medicaid. Yeah, it's really complicated; they [Medicaid] will reject anything if they can.[15]

Case management services are a vital part of supportive housing and Housing First. This administrative barrier presents a direct challenge to supportive housing policy by placing high barriers to retaining critical services.

Beyond direct billing, Medicaid networks present a similar challenge for local community organizations working to address homelessness and chronic homelessness. Despite Medicaid expansion, interviewees cited challenges finding providers who accept Medicaid, especially in the realm of primary care. This challenge compounds the effects of an environment already rife with implementation barriers. The compounding effect happens by constricting service access for at-risk clients who require medical interventions and coordinated primary care to manage and ameliorate homelessness (Stergiopoulos et al. 2015). Interviewees cited the limited Medicaid provider networks to be products of the challenging funding environment, where providers may be disincentivized from accepting Medicaid as a payer due to administrative reimbursement challenges and low reimbursement rates. Ultimately, the misalignment between state-level administrative requirements governing billing practices and shaping provider networks creates additional administrative burdens for practitioners on the ground. These administrative burdens ultimately influence practitioners' ability to adequately implement supportive housing policy and programming and homelessness services overall.

Second, interviewees described administrative implementation barriers arising from policy misalignment over issues inherent to homelessness. Interviewees described challenges illustrating a lack of alignment between Medicaid policy procedures and Medicaid's ability to work with and address the needs of persons experiencing homelessness, despite the high target population overlap between Medicaid recipients and homeless and chronically homeless individuals. The two most common examples of this type of policy misalignment interviewees cited are the relationship between homelessness and incarceration and the administrative burden of Medicaid enrollment for individuals experiencing homelessness.

The policy implementation challenges stemming from the interactions of incarceration, homelessness, and Medicaid are very similar to the challenges facing San Francisco. Because of the strong relationship between incarceration and homelessness (Ware and Dennis 2013), individuals experiencing chronic homelessness tend to cycle in and out of jail. This cycling often leads to gaps in services for individuals released from incarceration and is associated with higher rates of homelessness upon re-entry, especially for individuals who were homeless prior to incarceration (McNiel, Binder, and Robinson 2005). In Shreveport specifically, interviewees stated that over half of incarcerated individuals in local jails are formerly homeless or cycling in and out of jail and homelessness (HOPE Connections 2003; Hope for the Homeless 2014). Local data were not available to verify these estimates, but a point-in-time count from Louisiana in 2013 showed 40% of homeless individuals surveyed had been recently incarcerated (Matheny et al. 2013, 19). Medicaid enrollment does not work well in practice to address the persistent relationship between homelessness and incarceration (Snyder 2016; Medicaid Reentry Act, 2019). Therefore, when individuals experiencing homelessness who are enrolled in Medicaid are incarcerated, they lose Medicaid (Louisiana Department of Health 2017b, 4) and are often not re-enrolled upon re-entry (Medicaid and CHIP Payment and Access Commission 2018, 5; Council of State Governments 2013). The Louisiana Department of Health (2017a) is working to address this policy misalignment, which may in the future reduce coverage gaps and enrollment challenges.

This persistent service gap further perpetuates homelessness after re-entry by not promoting access to crucial services that can help reduce homelessness and manage chronic medical and behavioral health conditions (Greenberg and Rosenheck 2008; Hawthorne et al. 2012). The policy misalignment between Medicaid enrollment and outreach in Louisiana and the lived experience of individuals experiencing chronic homelessness in Shreveport creates inherent barriers to effective supportive housing and homeless policy implementation by perpetuating gaps in access to necessary services (U.S. Department of Health and Human Services Assistant Secretary for Planning and Evaluation and Office of Disability Aging and Long-Term Care Policy 2018).

> I have been to several meetings with the Louisiana LaPre program, which is a special pilot program for post incarceration. I have tried to stress the importance of providing RX & patient info about the person being released so they can provide that info to us when they return to the community. Unfortunately, we still have folks show up at [our clinic], with five days of meds [that are put in a brown paper envelope] and they have no written medical or RX documentation. That is how they are released. It makes more difficult for us to continue with care.[16]

Enrollment procedures and eligibility requirements also create inherent barriers to supportive housing and homelessness policy and programming overall by not tailoring policy approaches to population specific needs. Interviewees discussed two main administrative barriers related to Medicaid enrollment and eligibility. As discussed in Chapter 5 of this volume on San Francisco, prior to Medicaid expansion the majority of chronically homeless individuals were not eligible for Medicaid (Warfield, DiPietro, and Artiga 2016). This new eligibility has been a big benefit to individuals experiencing homelessness in Shreveport. What has been a challenge is the administrative process of enrolling in Medicaid individuals experiencing homelessness, as well as the eligibility requirements outlined by Medicaid that do not align with needs or reality of homelessness.

Interviewees cited enrollment procedures as a common administrative barrier that created policy implementation conflict as a result of direct discord from issues inherent to homelessness. These enrollment procedures are common among federal medical and social service benefit programs. However, these requirements create policy trade-offs for actors in the policy space as a result of the benefit inaccessibility for their targeted population.

In Shreveport, interviewees cited basic enrollment procedures, including having a form of identification, as barriers to Medicaid enrollment for persons experiencing long-term homelessness. Often, such individuals have been without formal identification or any kind of identification for a very long period of time. Thus, requiring formal identification may create a barrier due to lack of trust among this vulnerable population, as well as through the processes required to obtain formal identification itself. As a result, provider organizations both in the Continuum of Care and external to the Continuum of Care face a choice of either providing in-house identification and enrollment processes or not offering or relying on Medicaid resources due to these multiple levels of enrollment barriers persons experiencing chronic homelessness and severe poverty endure.

> For homeless folks, getting IDs and paperwork to enroll in Medicaid can be a challenge at times. Some of the homeless providers, who say they help with IDs don't provide a good service all the time.[17]
> Before [Medicaid expansion] we had charity hospitals, there was no need for any documentation of any kind, that is . . . it was easier for super poor people, for working poor or people like that [to get care].[18]

The reality of this trade-off exemplifies the misalignment between local- and state-level policy mechanisms in design and implementation ultimately limits successful public policy alternatives targeting homelessness, which shapes access to services for individuals experiencing chronic homelessness.

The disconnect between the reality of homelessness and Medicaid eligibility also generates more challenges for homeless policy and programming in Shreveport. Shreveport is a municipality that exists 30 minutes outside of the Texas border. As mentioned in Atlanta and San Francisco, persons experiencing homelessness, especially chronic homelessness, are often mobile within or between metropolitan areas (Gray et al. 2011). Due to the proximity with Texas, many persons experiencing homelessness in Shreveport have often moved from Texas or move between Texas and Louisiana. This mobility creates fundamental challenges for Medicaid eligibility since eligibility is tied directly to an individual's place of residence, specifically parish (county) and state (State Health Access Data Assistance Center, Division of Health Policy and Management, and University of Minnesota School of Public Health 2018).

Since persons experiencing homelessness do not have a place of residence, this policy misalignment between Medicaid and homeless needs creates consistent barriers to policy implementation. The barriers to policy implementation are generated by reducing accessibility to medical and other supportive services necessary to address the causes of chronic homelessness. In effect, when persons move to Shreveport from Texas and are on Texas Medicaid, they cannot receive services, and either must go back to Texas or must re-enroll in Louisiana Medicaid.

> People will be coming in from Texas and Arkansas, they get on the bus, they have Texas Medicaid, but they can't get their Medication filled, we get them enrolled in Louisiana Medicaid until they complete that process, or they can leave again.[19]

Similarly, when persons live across parish lines in off-grid areas, residency is difficult to determine. Or, if individuals move between parishes as a result of police responses or service needs, they may not be able to access services outside of their parish network based on their Medicaid eligibility network.

Funding Constraints

Funding was the second major concern or barrier interviewees discussed in reference to the role of state policies in shaping local homelessness policy and programming. Interviewees broadly emphasized that the State of Louisiana was not involved or was involved to a lesser degree compared to local and federal counterparts. Medicaid was the policy referenced most often by interviewees as a source of funding with constraints. However, interviewees reiterated an overall concern for the lack of state involvement or funding for behavioral health services and supportive services for homelessness programming generally from any state entity. Effectively, the interviews demonstrated a state policy space that both (1) runs parallel to local homeless policy interests but due to misaligned interests or funding constraints is not able to interact effectively with local priorities, while simultaneously illustrating a state-level policy space that is (2) otherwise absent due to greater economic constraints on the State of Louisiana. The misaligned interests between state and local policy or funding constraints have negative consequences for homeless policy by creating a state policy space that does not directly address the complex needs of persons experience homelessness, despite the high degree of Medicaid enrollment by persons experiencing homelessness.

When thinking about local-level incentives for supportive housing policy, actors consistently referenced state-level policies that exist that could be leveraged for supportive housing policy but are unable due either to state and local policy misalignment or to overall funding constraints within these state-level policies. Considering the first issue of policy misalignment, the majority of actors in Shreveport expressed concerns similar to those in San Francisco. This is the fact that Medicaid policy is a great resource for health services but has significant funding limitations for anything beyond the scope of traditional health services. This illustrates a fundamental policy misalignment. Medicaid is increasingly advertised as a policy space amenable to homelessness programming, specifically in the context of supportive housing policy. However, Medicaid does not currently pay for housing itself (Paradise and Cohen Ross 2017).

Further, local actors face many barriers to leveraging Medicaid resources for other supportive services beyond housing, too. The supportive services that nearly all interviewees mentioned as outside of current state policy resources are long-term behavioral health services. All health providers interviewed independently cited limited funding for long-term behavioral health services, even with Medicaid expansion.

> No one is taking homeless people who are mentally ill. Nowhere for them to go.
> I deal with this weekly. Twice a month, I get a call from a parent, 20 years old,
> schizophrenic, homeless, nowhere to go. No funding for long-term care.[20]

Louisiana currently has multiple Medicaid 1915c waivers to be used for long-term behavioral health services through permanent supportive housing (PSH) among various at-risk populations (Centers for Medicare and Medicaid Services 2019; Wagner 2017). However, in 2017 Louisiana only had just over 2,000 PSH units available for the entire state (Wagner 2017). Further, state-level policy documents outline presumed coordination between state-level Medicaid policy and the Louisiana Housing Authority to develop and implement PSH among chronically homeless populations (Department of Health 2017; Wagner 2017). The lack of knowledge among interviewees of state-level PSH activity for long-term behavioral health services paired with state acknowledgment of limited capacity and coordination challenges suggests that findings of policy misalignment between state and local government may be occurring at the implementation phase. The misalignment may be a product of the fact that Louisiana's efforts to target long-term behavioral health among this population are relatively new, as well as the fact that coordination challenges between traditional "health services", Medicaid policy, and housing policy may further compound effects of misalignment by attempting to merge two programs with very different goals and administrative mechanisms.

The recent efforts by Louisiana to merge the state policy administrative entities coordinating housing and supportive services for persons experiencing chronic homelessness may signal downstream policy change that would increase alignment of policy goals across the state and local policy efforts to eventually improve supportive housing policy implementation (Department of Health 2017; Wagner 2017). However, an ongoing concern that may threaten these efforts is the limited capacity in terms of funding and housing output (units) for supportive housing development, even with ongoing state efforts (Department of Health 2017). Interviewees additionally discussed the presence of the Louisiana Housing Corporation as a great coordinator of federal funding, but with limited funding opportunities overall (Louisiana Housing Corporation 2016, 3).

Concerns about funding limitations in general, beyond issues of policy misalignment, take us to the second major finding regarding state involvement and funding. Interviewees discussed the increasingly uncertain economic circumstances facing Louisiana as a state. Interviewees often connected notions about state economic disadvantage to limited or absent state funding overall, as well as a reliance among policy makers and providers in the homeless policy space on federal funding and nonprofit donations over state resources as a whole.

> You have to understand our state is a very depressed condition right now economically, facing really challenging financial cuts last few years, that has severely limited what the state can do. . . . I don't think they have the resources or finances to really do what would be ideal. I just don't think the state can become the player it could be or should be just because of those constraints.[21]

The majority of interviewees stressed Louisiana's dire economic situation in the context of any state involvement in homelessness policy or programming or tangential policies. Interviewees, including all state employees who were interviewed, felt that Louisiana's economic circumstances constrained state-level grants or investments in this policy space as well as others. Interviewees felt that these limitations constrained Louisiana to the degree that even without any political constraints the state could not become more involved in homelessness policy due to economic concerns. These concerns reiterate the potential for capacity constraints to limit state involvement in homelessness policy and programing even in the face of policy alignment efforts.

Unlike San Francisco and Atlanta, Shreveport serves as the representative case for municipalities without a local government-level supportive housing policy. Shreveport is a case where the Continuum of Care and municipal policy goals, decision-making, and implementation remain very separate. The separation is evident in policy decision-making and implementation, where the municipality has little to no involvement in homeless policy aside from coordinating pass-through federal funding. The Continuum of Care operates independently, debating homeless policy choices and implementing policies without aid and little to no input from the local government. The lack of involvement by Shreveport's municipal government presents direct barriers to supportive housing policy design and implementation in Shreveport, by restricting the authority and the resources available to the Continuum of Care to coordinate policy activities.

Unlike Atlanta and San Francisco, where the local government and the Continuum of Care have merged to jointly govern homeless policy, the Shreveport Continuum of Care remains independent, and this independence effectively constrains its ability to design and implement some policy changes. As discussed in the chapter, policing remains a persistent challenge in interactions with persons experiencing chronic homelessness, as well as a challenge for federal requirements to move away from punitive policing responses to homelessness and chronic homelessness. Since the Continuum of Care has no municipal authority, it is greatly limited in its ability to coordinate with the Shreveport Police Department, to require trainings on best practices or responses to individuals experiencing chronic homelessness and SMI, or support coordinated entry practices with the assistance of police officers. Zoning remains another challenge. With limited ability to participate in municipal debates, the Continuum of Care is often disadvantaged in debates over new shelter or low-income housing constructions and often overshadowed by economic elites in the DDA. This is a stark comparison to San Francisco, and even Atlanta, where Continuum of Care actors are a part of the municipal bureaucracy, are heavily involved in policy design with city officials, and are able to coordinate with and facilitate design and implementation of policing interventions, supportive housing policy design and development, and municipal-level funding initiatives.

The Continuum of Care in Shreveport is a very strong organization with actors who have substantial policy expertise and have been able to design a coordinated entry approach that embraces Housing First. The Continuum of Care has been able to develop these activities due to strong buy-in from the local Continuum of Care stakeholder network, even in the face of limited municipal support. If the Continuum of Care did have a formal municipal role, their existing policy capacity would place them in a solid position to lobby for policing and re-entry interventions, more supportive housing units and shelter development, and possibly municipal revenue sources to fill in existing resource gaps. Without a formal role for Continuum of Care actors, most of these activities may remain voluntary—hinging on the interest from other actors with few incentives to participate—constraining public policy alternatives for Shreveport and other city cases of strong homeless policy devolution and decentralization.

CHAPTER 8

A Way Forward

UNUSUAL SUSPECTS: CONTINUUMS OF CARE AND MUNICIPAL SOLUTIONS TO CHRONIC HOMELESSNESS

Chronic homelessness has severe implications for health disparities. Black Americans are four times and Hispanic Americans are two times more likely to experience homelessness compared to white Americans (Fusaro, Levy, and Shaefer 2018). Homelessness contributes to high rates of chronic disease, adverse behavioral health outcomes, increased mortality, and lower rates of educational and job attainment over the life course (U.S. Interagency Council on Homelessness 2015). Longer durations of homelessness are associated with higher mortality rates, adverse behavioral health outcomes, and chronic medical conditions; moreover, persons experiencing chronic homelessness are more likely to remain homeless as length of homelessness increases (Stafford and Wood 2017). Homelessness and chronic homelessness hit large metropolitan areas especially hard over the past two decades (U.S. Department of Housing and Urban Development 2018g). Unsheltered homelessness, which is primarily long-term homelessness, is increasing again for the first time in 10 years. What are municipalities doing to address this public health crisis?

Homelessness is a surprising case of a public health issue that is governed by a primarily decentralized system of nongovernmental actors—both historically and today. The history of devolution and decentralization in homelessness governance makes it a unique policy arena where various actors compete and implement very different types of policies, all attempting to manage homelessness and long-term homelessness to different ends. The U.S. Department of Housing and Urban Development has recently

Ungoverned and Out of Sight. Charley E. Willison, Oxford University Press (2021). © Oxford University Press.
DOI: 10.1093/oso/9780197548325.003.0008

been encouraging partnerships between nongovernmental actors and local governments in homeless policy governance to help improve policy coordination and implementation. This book specifically investigates why municipal governments approach solutions to chronic homelessness in different ways, and, as this research emphasized, why municipal governments may get involved in solutions to address chronic homelessness at all, when local governments have historically been minor players in a major problem for U.S. cities.

Most research on homelessness focuses on empirical research identifying best practices for solutions to chronic or long-term homelessness. However, there is a wide gap in the literature investigating the political processes shaping the reality of establishing or implementing these best practices. This book seeks to understand the political processes influencing adoption of best-practice solutions to reduce chronic homelessness, or homeless policy decision-making, in municipalities across the United States.

This book argues that homelessness policy is a very fragmented and disjointed policy space as a result of decades of decentralization. Responses to chronic homelessness are governed in four separate and distinct policy arenas: the state, local government, economic elites or the economically powerful in municipalities, and homeless service providers or the Continuum of Care.[1] The separation and conflict between these governing approaches result in increased challenges to establishing and implementing effective policy solutions to end chronic homelessness. Challenges include relatively limited state-level support such as financial resources and/or administrative burdens stemming from misaligned policy goals between state policies and Continuum of Care programming or the needs of persons experiencing homelessness on the ground; inequity in political participation that may exclude at-risk populations or bias participation in favor of economic elites; and, finally, limited involvement by municipal governments in many cases. When municipal governments remain absent from homeless governance, Continuums of Care may be constrained in their ability to carry out policies and programming as a result of insufficient funding and coordinate with local government other necessary services such as behavioral healthcare, Medicaid administration, policing and incarceration, and zoning for or construction of supportive housing units themselves. Ultimately, conflicting policy goals across the four policy arenas and decentralization of homelessness policy governance contribute to fewer evidence-based, publicly funded policy alternatives for solutions to chronic homelessness and increase the policy alternatives for private actors(here, economic elites).

This research finds that growth in policy capacity paired with structural changes incentivizing recentralization of homelessness governance may be required to promote interaction and coordination across the policy approaches to overcome collective action problems and develop and implement effective solutions to long-term homelessness. However, a persistent problem that may require solutions beyond integration of the Continuum of Care and municipal government are protections of minority group and policy target populations in homeless policy debates. Across all cases in the research, homeless policy decision-making typically excludes persons who are at risk of, currently, or formerly homeless. This bias in policy decision-making may promote implementation challenges by skewing processes in favor of elite preferences who generally oppose permanent supportive housing and may lead to policy adoption that does not successfully address the causes of chronic homelessness. This chapter reviews the primary findings from the results of the research and subsequently provides recommendations for policy makers to improve homeless policy governance systems to design and deliver policies that successfully ameliorate chronic homelessness.

A WAY FORWARD: THEORETICAL AND POLICY CONTRIBUTIONS

Overall, six main themes arise from this research that help us explain why municipalities approach solutions to chronic homelessness in different ways and why municipalities may or may not use evidence-based strategies (i.e., supportive housing or Housing First).[2] These main findings align with the overall argument of the book: *decentralization* and a *fragmented* policy space contribute to more policy alternatives for private actors and fewer policy alternatives for publicly funded, evidence-based policy efforts.

This section discusses the theoretical and policy implications of these main findings and offers policy recommendations for each to improve local homeless policy decision-making and implementation in U.S. municipalities, going forward: (1) the implications of delegating a public health policy space to nongovernmental actors and how it works in practice; (2) the growth of policy capacity as an important step in building a municipal, governmental response to homelessness beyond solely delegated state actors; (3) the role of institutional restructuring in overlapping policy areas as an incentive for municipal governmental buy-in to formally participate in solutions to chronic homelessness; (4) the role of municipal fragmentation in exacerbating challenges in homeless policy decision-making and implementation; (5) the role of the social construction of homelessness in competing policy approaches to chronic homelessness pursued by economic elites; and (6) the implications of misaligned state policies, especially for state-level policies intended to assist persons experiencing chronic homelessness or that directly target needs of persons experiencing chronic homelessness.

Solutions for a Delegated State

Delegation and Authority

First, this research is a case study of the functioning of the delegated state[3] as a main public health policy delivery system. Previous research on the delegated state has focused on defining and describing the submerged state, how it has changed over time, and its development. There are few studies of the implications of the submerged state as a *policy mechanism* in practice. This research helps to fill that gap. The literature that does exist on the functioning and consequences of the submerged or delegated state discusses the implications of delegation for democracy (Mettler 2011; Soss, Fording, and Schram 2011; Morgan and Campbell 2011). The findings in my research illustrate a similar, overall relationship. In the case studies, delegated state actors who are not integrated into formal municipal decision-making processes face participatory challenges (such as not being invited to municipal governmental meetings), relegating actors to their own, separate decision-making apparatus relying on inconsistent funding structures (grants and donations) and limited authority to implement policies they have designed (and no authority over other governmental institutions that may be crucial to supportive housing policy implementation such as policing, zoning, and municipal funding including taxation, municipal bonds, and intergovernmental transfers). In cases of complete delegation of homeless services governance to nongovernmental actors, as shown in the case of Shreveport, nongovernmental actors face constrained decision-making and implementation processes that limit the overall success of policies and programs aimed to reduce chronic homelessness. For example, Shreveport's Continuum of Care faced ongoing challenges with policing. Persons experiencing chronic homelessness were frequently fined or arrested for quality-of-life crimes, interrupting access to supportive homeless services. Continuum of Care actors offered trainings to the Police Department to improve responses to persons experiencing homelessness, especially persons with severe mental illness. However, Continuum of Care actors could only *request* police officers' compliance, as a result of no municipal regulatory authority for the Continuum of Care, making any reforms to policing responses to homelessness entirely voluntary.

Many Continuums of Care may disagree with these findings, arguing, along with many debates in federalism, that there are substantial trade-offs to decentralization, a primary benefit being the ability to tailor programming to local needs, without being held to specific funding priorities and requirements. Yet, as previously discussed and demonstrated in this book, there are many challenges and drawbacks to complete delegation to nongovernmental actors, much of which lies in limited authority to design and implement effective policy and programming, as a result of participatory inequity, limited policy capacity (i.e., funding and other resources), and institutional structures. In cases where Continuums of Care may remain fully decentralized, or not a part of municipal government, improving existing relationships with local governmental entities through various forms of formal coordination may help alleviate the challenges associated with decentralization.

Policy Capacity

The second main finding is the important role of policy capacity as a step in establishing a formal, municipal supportive housing policy. If the delegated state faces substantial constraints in policy decision-making and implementation as a result of their institutional organization, how do we move toward forma municipal involvement in supportive housing policy? Atlanta and San Francisco suggest that municipal-level investment in policy capacity—systems and/or resources including funding sufficient to respond to chronic homelessness and associated problems—may be a crucial part of the process for establishing a municipal governmental supportive housing policy by *generating capacity* of municipal governments to be able to respond to and effectively participate in supportive housing policy. Historically, and in contemporary cases that rely on complete delegation (e.g., Shreveport), policy capacity to address chronic homelessness and homelessness overall resided with the Continuums of Care, or this governance system of nongovernmental actors, primarily nonprofit organizations. If the entire system is decentralized and authority is delegated to this decentralized system, it may be unlikely that cities or counties may have sufficient resources to be able to adequately participate in homeless policy governance without establishing some kind of policy capacity of their own. Resource investment may be especially important but more difficult for lower-income municipalities, where local governments may rely more on state, federal, and philanthropic funding for social services than municipal sources (Hajnal and Trounstine 2010).

Atlanta and San Francisco both document a long build-up over many years of municipal investment in resources—staffing and funding—to address chronic homelessness and problems related to chronic homelessness (e.g., HIV/AIDS and behavioral health) prior to discussions about a municipal governmental role in addressing homelessness and chronic homelessness. As discussed, the city of Shreveport did not make similar resource investments of any kind. Theoretically, it makes sense that recentralization of homeless policy governance would possibly necessitate this resource investment. Otherwise municipalities face a trade-off between insufficient means to govern homeless policy at the municipal level and continued delegation to the existing systems where policy capacity lies—the delegated state, or the Continuum of Care.

Institutional Restructuring

The third finding posits the relationship between existing institutional arrangements and a formal municipal role in homeless policy governance. In both San Francisco and Atlanta, the shift toward a municipal supportive housing policy and the local Continuum of Care becoming integrated into municipal government was anteceded not only by notable amounts of funding and other resources but also by a shift in the municipal role governing other similar policy spaces related to chronic homelessness. In San Francisco, administration of behavioral healthcare shifted from the State of California, acting as a pass-through funding agency to mostly community-based organizations providing outpatient care at the local level to county governments. This shift, while on its face is decentralization, had the effect of recentralizing behavioral healthcare at the local level by shifting policy implementation to county governments rather than nongovernmental, mostly private community-based organizations and providing counties the responsibility to design, regulate, and monitor community-based care (Penner 1995, 275, 280; Snowden, Scheffler, and Zhang 2002). This reform making counties the arbiters of care for persons with severe mental illness, many of whom were homeless, spurred discussions about governmental responsibility for persons experiencing homelessness.

In Atlanta, governance of the local Continuum of Care moved from a joint-governance arrangement across three counties in the Atlanta metropolitan area—DeKalb County, Fulton County, and the City of Atlanta—to three separate Continuums of Care to receive more federal funding for each local jurisdiction. The decision to separate the trijurisdiction Continuum of Care forced the City of Atlanta to choose how the new Continuum would be governed. The primary question was whether or not the City of Atlanta would have an informal governance role, as it was previously, delegating governance to nonprofit providers, or whether the city would introduce a formal governance role.

In Atlanta and San Francisco, both decisions to formalize municipal governance of homeless policy and subsequently *adopt* a municipal supportive housing policy occurred after not only these institutional realignments but also after years of substantial investment in financing and local expertise to directly address homelessness and chronic homelessness. Like policy capacity, the role of institutional reconfigurations in municipal choices to formalize homeless policy governance makes sense at first glance. These institutional shifts may have provided a window of opportunity for policy change, likely conditional on existing municipal policy capacity, that allowed municipalities to act where they may have otherwise not had the ability or incentives to do so, especially given strong path dependence of delegation to nongovernmental actors. Further research is needed to understand the prevalence of institutional shifts in incentivizing municipal homeless policy governance. For policy makers, this finding may not represent a necessary condition, but may be a relevant factor when considering homeless policy decision-making.

Solutions for a Fragmented Policy Space

Municipal Fragmentation

The fourth finding and policy recommendation pertain to the challenges associated with overlapping jurisdictions for implementing supportive housing policy. Atlanta is a case study in the realities of the challenges associated with multiple, overlapping municipal jurisdictions in attempting to coordinate policies that necessitate collective action. The challenges Atlanta faces are certainly not unique to the Atlanta metropolitan area. Los Angeles, one of the largest cities in the United Sates with the highest rates of homelessness and chronic homelessness, has 89 separate jurisdictions within the county of Los Angeles (U.S. Census Bureau 2012). What the findings from Atlanta demonstrate, are that these multiple, overlapping municipal jurisdictions create challenges for supportive housing policy in two ways: (1) by promoting gatekeeping mechanisms by economic elites or the economically powerful to protect their neighborhoods from supportive housing development and utilizing reactionary policing policies against persons experiencing chronic homelessness and (2) by constraining Continuums of Care ability to successfully coordinate various supportive housing policy components—including counts of homelessness and coordinated entry (process to screen individuals and distribute services based on vulnerability; U.S. Department of Housing and Urban Development 2015a)—across various jurisdictions that may vary in their levels of engagement.

However, this research cannot fully explain *why* economic elites, who employ gatekeeping mechanisms to oppose supportive housing development and reactionary policies that leverage policing to remove persons experiencing chronic homelessness from their neighborhoods, engage in policies aligned with the *individual* social construction of homelessness (e.g., whether it is a product of existing social construction and/or for their own political or economic gains). This notion targets undesirable behaviors associated with homelessness, or behaviors that have been historically associated with "individual failings." Policies targeting individual failings conflict with policies seeking to address the *causes* of chronic homelessness—which necessitate upstream investments in housing and medical care—or supportive housing and Housing First.

As illustrated in San Francisco and Shreveport, economic elites utilize this paradigm to approach chronic homelessness even in jurisdictions with far less municipal fragmentation. The challenge with municipal fragmentation and reactionary approaches to chronic homelessness is that the power of elites is exacerbated, by institutionally protected neighborhoods. As shown in Atlanta, elites leverage policing to move persons experiencing chronic homelessness to the boundaries *between* jurisdictions where they are less visible, as a result of the strong opposition from protected neighborhoods in those jurisdictions. Restrictive zoning arrangements within county jurisdictions presents further challenges to supportive housing construction. Los Angeles and other highly fragmented metropolitan areas may experience similar challenges, where white, wealthy jurisdictions may have a disproportionate, collective influence on the population of persons experiencing chronic homelessness in the county overall.

Continuums of Care, or homeless policy governance structures, encounter challenges related to municipal fragmentation, too. As Atlanta shows, the Continuum of Care, even when it exists as a part of municipal government, exists in a metropolitan area seeking policy solutions to the *same* population, across the multiple, overlapping municipal jurisdictions. To this end, coordination is required across all jurisdictions to promote successful supportive housing policy implementation. Without it, authority and responsibility for different populations across jurisdictions and between them becomes unclear, and some jurisdictions may shirk responsibilities to the detriment of the larger policy goals. Formalizing accountability and transparency mechanisms between jurisdictions may improve participation and coordination. In addition, formalizing engagement by municipal governments in homeless policy governance may help improve transparency and accountability—for example, in cases where some Continuums of Care across jurisdictions may not be a part of municipal government, possibly constraining participation and oversight.

Social Construction

The fifth finding and policy point clearly align with the fourth. As discussed, social constructions of persons experiencing chronic homelessness, when informing responses to homelessness, can be exacerbated in fragmented municipal environments. Yet, even without municipal fragmentation, informal policies adhering to individual explanations of homelessness produce policies that directly conflict with supportive housing policy success by interfering with bureaucratic expertise, initiating reactionary policing as an informal policy mechanism toward persons experiencing chronic homelessness and generating entrenched opposition to supportive housing construction itself. Overall, while all of these policies focus on addressing the *visibility* of homelessness as opposed to the causes of homelessness, these informal policies have one other aspect in common as discussed in San Francisco and Atlanta: bias toward economic elites in policy processes.

In each of these instances—interfering with bureaucratic tasks, leveraging police responses, or opposing new housing construction—economic elites, whether organized, corporate interests, or groups of wealthy neighbors, comprise the majority of the stakeholders in the debates or policy mechanisms. This limited representation biases policy processes toward elite interests, by obscuring representation from other groups, including groups at the crux of the policies in question: persons at risk of, currently, or formerly homeless. While there are many challenges associated with improving participation by at-risk groups, including time and fiscal constraints individuals face, some organizations have managed to do so. The Board of Directors for Boston Health Care for the Homeless is partially comprised of and includes board seats for persons with lived experience of homelessness, who additionally sit on a consumer advisory board for the organization (Boston Health Care for the Homeless Program 2020). Community Development Block Grant funding requires community participation and engagement to protect underrepresented groups from further marginalization (U.S. Department of Housing and Urban Development 2014). Yet most housing policy debates currently consist of economic elites opposing housing construction (Einstein, Palmer, and Glick 2018, 2019). Mechanisms to improve representation and participation by at-risk groups and persons with lived experience of homelessness will help reduce bias in supportive housing policy debates. Reforming political processes to institutionalize or require participation by at-risk groups in policy debates can protect against elite bias and protect minority group representation.

Instances of elite bias in policing and bureaucratic policymaking may be reduced by improving accountability mechanisms. Many large municipalities, as discussed in San Francisco, make 311 data documenting police responses to persons experiencing homelessness public. San Francisco also, as discussed in Chapter 5 of this volume, has a regulatory response to chronic homelessness and policing, by developing a trained Homeless Outreach Team within policing to help improve police relations with persons experiencing chronic homelessness. Despite this, as San Francisco illustrates, relations have not improved. One challenge is that the upstream factor influencing these police responses are requests initiated by economic elites—in the case of San Francisco, wealthy homeowners and in the cases of Atlanta and Shreveport, organized businesses interests within the city. Improved accountability mechanisms to regulate elite uses of policing against persons experiencing homelessness is one option. San Francisco recently proposed legislation to make it illegal for individuals to make racially motivated police calls or calls against persons who are doing nothing wrong but have the police called on them as a result of their race (A. Bauman 2020). San Francisco also recently announced that they will reduce police responses to homelessness for noncriminal, or quality-of-life calls, similar to the pilot project in Atlanta (Dolan 2020). This is an important first step, and replacing police officers with trained first medical and social service responders may have a measurable influence (A. V. Smith 2020). However, as shown in Atlanta, until the program is implemented widely, or well enforced bureaucratically, existing challenges may remain. Despite the additional mechanism of banning calls to the police—from civilians or organizations—against persons experiencing chronic homelessness for quality-of-life issues, the upstream, informal police mechanisms may persist.

Bringing the State Back In

Last is the theme of misaligned state policies, in particular policies intended to address problems associated with chronic homelessness. While there are many different state policies, Medicaid expansion was the primary focus of interviewees, given the scope of Medicaid services that are relevant for addressing chronic homelessness and the absence of other state level policies and a historical state-level role in homeless policy overall. Other state policies pertain to funding—the utilization of which is often conditional on local policy processes that, as shown in San Francisco, are often intercepted by economic elites and require improved representation in local homeless policy debates. Regardless, additional state-level funding for local supportive housing policy may prove vitally important in municipalities with local funding constraints to circumvent federal funding shortages, as shown in Atlanta and Shreveport.

Health policy has often championed Medicaid expansion as a silver bullet policy, solving problems of access to healthcare for low-income persons. And this research does show that Medicaid expansion has certainly benefited persons experiencing chronic homelessness by expanding eligibility levels to include single adults. However, this research demonstrates the practical realities of Medicaid expansion implementation for this at-risk population. Shreveport and San Francisco both illustrate enrollment challenges associated with Medicaid administrative procedures, despite divergent governance arrangements.

As a border city in Louisiana, Shreveport receives many persons experiencing homelessness from Texas. When persons arrive from Texas in Louisiana, they must be re-enrolled in Louisiana Medicaid before they can receive care. In California, county-level administration of Medicaid has caused challenges for enrollment and care access in San Francisco. Individuals experiencing chronic homelessness move within municipal jurisdictions in the Bay Area. When individuals move between counties, such as Oakland and San Francisco, providers have to identify county residence and often re-enroll persons based on the county they are currently seeking care in. Medicaid administration does not align with the reality of the transient nature of chronic homelessness and creates challenges for care access and care coordination. Similar problems arise related to the strong relationship between incarceration and chronic homelessness. In both Shreveport and San Francisco, providers face continual disenrollment challenges as a result of incarceration. Often, persons are not reconnected with services or re-enrolled in Medicaid after re-entry. This is another example of how the practical application of Medicaid expansion is more complex and may not work well for certain, highly vulnerable populations.

These persistent challenges illustrated in San Francisco and Shreveport emphasize the importance of coordination between different policies and the different levels of government that serve the same population. Centralization of the Continuum of Care in municipal government is not enough to prevent fragmented policy goals and divergent implementation processes across intergovernmental relations. Greater alignment between Medicaid administration and local, population-specific needs may help alleviate some of these implementation challenges and increase the opportunities for supportive housing policy success.

Recommendations to improve policy alignment include promoting greater coordination and centralization of homeless policy governance at the municipal level to allow policies to coordinate more effectively with other public health and state-level programs (Rosenbaum et al. 2016), such as county Medicaid agencies. Recommendations to alleviate functional challenges of Medicaid access in homeless policy arise from aligning Medicaid policy with the needs of persons experiencing chronic homelessness. This includes creating alternatives to residential eligibility requirements as most homeless individuals are transient or without addresses. An alternative recommendation includes transitioning to state as opposed to county-level administration to reduce re-enrollment associated with county-level administration. Relatedly, Medicaid can permit long-term enrollment to reduce the chance that an individual will lose coverage based on failure to re-enroll. Other recommendations include improving service coordination during re-entry from incarceration and expanding the services that Medicaid may finance, including housing. To achieve these goals and improve access to services and health outcomes for individuals experiencing chronic homelessness, those involved in Medicaid expansion and homeless policy efforts must coordinate their efforts and adopt strategies that address the barriers particular to this population.

CONCLUSION

Addressing chronic homelessness is an ongoing challenge for municipalities across the United States. This research presents a picture of a policy space that requires interaction between different policy sectors yet has been broadly left out of the scope of existing policies and institutionally omitted from policy processes. The result is a need to work backwards to institutionalize homeless policy governance and solutions to chronic homelessness in formal policy processes to give policy makers and advocates an even playing field with other sectors of public health and social policy. This includes formalizing Continuums' of Care relationships with municipal government to provide them sufficient authority to and capacity to carry out policy tasks and thus formally aligning necessary policy coordination for supportive housing policy efforts with public health, housing, policing, and Medicaid, among others. Until issues of authority can be remedied for homeless policy governance systems and, subsequently, issues of fragmentation across competing or misaligned policy spaces are addressed through improved coordination, representation, and oversight, publicly funded, evidence-based policy solutions to chronic homelessness at the systems level may continue to flounder.

Data Set Overview and Codebook

The data set is comprised of 232 municipalities of 354 municipal Continuums of Care (CoCs) from the HUD 2016 Continuum of Care database to control for cities directly receiving federal homeless funding. The final sample accounts for 66% of all Continuums of Care in the United States. Municipalities were chosen based on their inclusion in the HUD 2016 Point-in-Time count survey, therefore selecting municipalities with a Continuum of Care that is receiving federal funding for homelessness solutions.

It is important to define "municipality" as measured, here. Municipalities, broadly, refer to units of local government including cities and or counties. This research purposefully does not choose between cities and counties in this data set but instead identifies the unit of analysis as local government jurisdictions existing within Continuums of Care that are primarily organized at the municipal level (e.g., one Continuum of Care in one city/county unit). In the data set, 208 Continuums of Care are contiguous with single-county borders. For 24 Continuums of Care covering more than one county, the largest county and aligning city was used as the unit of analysis.

There were 402 Continuums of Care in the United States in 2016. This data set includes all major city Continuums of Care, totaling 48 (e.g., San Francisco, Chicago, Boston) and 60% of all other Continuums of Care including small city and county Continuums of Care. Forty-eight regional, state, and U.S. territory Continuums of Care were dropped because these Continuums of Care are not aligned with specific municipalities and therefore cannot be used to evaluate municipal policy preferences. Small city and county Continuums of Care, totaling 124, were dropped due to a lack of municipal level data, including fiscal, population demographics, and political institutions. The final data set includes 232 municipal Continuums of Care, or 66% of all Continuums of Care in the United States.

CODEBOOK FSQCA/STATA CONVERSION PROCESS FOR QUANTITATIVE VARIABLES

Table A.1 FSQCA/STATA CONVERSION PROCESS FOR DEPENDENT VARIABLE

Dependent Variable	FSQCA Conversion	Data Source	Stata Conversion
Local governmental level of supportive housing policy	(1–0 [yes/no] for supportive housing policy)	Municipal supportive housing policies were collected from a search of city and county government websites, and Municode. A municipal policy was coded as "supportive housing" if a locality has one or more of the following: municipal plan(s), guidelines, regulations and or statutes establishing supportive housing, permanent supportive housing, and/ or Housing-First as the local government's approach to chronic homelessness.	(1–0 [yes/no] for supportive housing policy)

Table A.2 FSQCA/STATA CONVERSION PROCESS AND STATA CODEBOOK
FOR INDEPENDENT VARIABLES

Independent Variable	FSQCA Conversion (0–1)	Data Source	Stata Conversion
Continuum of Care type (municipal organization)	Major city COC = 1; smaller cities and counties = 0	U.S. Department of Housing and Urban Development (HUD; 2017c)	0/1; major city COC (1); smaller city, counties (0)
State or regional Continuum of Care	Statewide COC (Y/N); regional (0.5)	HUD (2017c)	0/1; statewide COC (1); regional (0.5)
Total homeless	1 = ≤10,000; 0.8 = 5,000–10,000; 0.6 = 1,000–5,000; 0.4 = 500–1,000; 0.2 = >500	HUD (2017c)	Discrete, numeric counts with no coded categories
Total chronically homeless	<1,000 = 1; 500–1,000 = 0.75; 250–500 = 0.5; 1–250 = 0.25	HUD (2017c)	Discrete, numeric counts with no coded categories
Total unsheltered chronically homeless	% of chronically homeless (decimal notation)	HUD (2017c)	Discrete, numeric counts with no coded categories
Total year-round permanent supportive housing beds	Included in the Stata analyses as an alternative measure of local supportive housing policy	HUD (2017c)	Discrete, numeric counts with no coded categories
Metropolitan statistical area (MSA) population	>1 million = 1; 250,000–1 million =0.75; 100,000–250,000 = 0.5, ≥100,000 = 0.25) (Census designation)	U.S. Census Bureau (2017)	Discrete, numeric counts with no coded categories
Gross domestic product (in current dollars) by MSA	>50,000 = 0.25; 50,000–100,000 = 0.5; 100,000–200,000 = 0.75; <200,000 = 1	Bureau of Economic Analysis (2017)	Discrete, numeric counts with no coded categories
Warm winter temperature	Used National Oceanic and Atmospheric Administration (NOAA) four-color categories of cold-warm; 0.25 = least warm winter temperature; 1.0 = warmest winter temperature	National Centers for Environmental Information and NOAA (2017)	Used NOAA four-color categories of cold-warm; 0.25 = least warm winter temperature; 1.0 = warmest winter temperature

(*continued*)

Independent Variable	FSQCA Conversion (0–1)	Data Source	Stata Conversion
Church-going population (public) (all denominations/ groups)	0/1 (1 = high); rates of adherence per 1,000 persons: 200–300 = 0.25; 300–400 = 0.35 . . . ; >800 = 1	Rates of adherence per 1,000 population; Association of Religion Data Archives (2010)	Rates of adherence per 1,000 persons; discrete, numeric counts with no coded categories
Southern region of the United States	0/1 (no/yes)	U.S. Department of Commerce Economics and Statistics Administration (2010)	0/1 (no/yes)
Former confederacy	0/1 (no/yes)	Editors of Encyclopaedia Britannica (2019)	0/1 (no/yes)
Sanctuary city federal U.S. Immigration and Customs Enforcement definition	Declined detainer: 0/1 (no/yes)	U.S. Immigrations and Customs Enforcement (2017)	Declined detainer: 0/1 (no/yes)
% white	Decimal notation	U.S. Census Bureau (2017)	Percentage of population identifying as white; discrete, numeric
% African American	Decimal notation	U.S. Census Bureau (2017)	Percentage of population identifying as Black; discrete, numeric
% Latino	Decimal notation	U.S. Census Bureau (2017)	Percent of population identifying as Latino; discrete, numeric
Total fragmentation	0–5 = 0.2; 6–15; 15–30 . . . >46 = 1	The total number of local governments in a county area; U.S. Census Bureau (2012b)	Discrete, numeric counts with no coded categories

Independent Variable	FSQCA Conversion (0–1)	Data Source	Stata Conversion
State Medicaid expansion	1/0 (yes/no)	National Conference of State Legislatures (2018)	1/0 (1 = expand; 0 = no)
State level supportive housing law or regulation	1/0 (yes/no)	State-level supportive housing policies were collected from a review of state government websites and Lexis-Nexis. States were coded using a binary measure of having a supportive housing policy or not (1/0) and coded as having a supportive-housing policy if the state had either a state plan, guideline, regulation, or statute establishing permanent supportive housing or Housing First was the state government's response approach to chronic homelessness	1/0 (yes/no)
Municipal institutional structure[a]	ICMA municipal form of government, 2011 data and definitions; plurality: 1 = most pluralistic form of government, 0 = least pluralistic; mayor council = 0.2 (least pluralistic); council manager = 0.4; commission = 0.6; town meeting = 0.8; representative town meeting = 0.1	International City/County Management Association (2011) Municipal Form of Government, 2011 Trends in Structure, Responsibility, and Composition	Retained International City/County Management Association codes for type of government: mayor council = 2; council manager = 4; commission = 6; town meeting = 8; representative town meeting = 1

(continued)

Independent Variable	FSQCA Conversion (0–1)	Data Source	Stata Conversion
MRP city policy conservatism (municipal ideology)	–1 to –0.4 = 0.25; –4 to 0 = 0.5; 0–0.2 = 0.75; >0.2 = 1; 1 = most conservative	Warshaw and Tausanovitch (2015)	Continuous; 0 = median; –1 = most liberal; 1 = most conservative
Concentration of nonprofit health organizations per capita	0–1 = low (0.1), 1–2 (0.2), 2–4 (0.35), 4–6 (0.55), 6–7 (0.75), ≥7 = high (1)	Per 10,000 people; National Center for Charitable Statistics (2018)	Discrete, numeric, rate per 10,000 ppl; no coded categories
Nonprofit health organizations per capita revenue	Maximum = 142,963.00; minimum = 0 (0 = 0; 1–1,000 = 0.1; 1001–2000 = 0.15; 2001–3000 = 0.25 . . . ≥10,000 = 1)	National Center for Charitable Statistics (2018)	Discrete, numeric counts with no coded categories
Private prisons (% prisoners in private prisons)	0 = 0; >10% = 0.25; ≤10% = 0.75; ≤20% = 1	U.S. Department of Justice. Office of Justice Programs (2011)	State-level data; discrete, numeric counts with no coded categories
Tourism	0 = 0; 1–1,000 = 0.1; 1001–2000 = 0.15; 2001–3000 = 0.25 . . . >10,000 = 1 (high)	Millions of dollars (arts, entertainment, recreation, accommodation, and food services), by Federal Information Processing Standard Publication MSA); Bureau of Economic Analysis (2017)	Millions of dollars by arts, entertainment categories; Discrete, numeric, no coded categories

[a]This measure was included in the initial analysis but dropped due to sample size constraints—the ICME data only aligned with 60 municipalities in the data set; initial results demonstrated that less pluralistic forms of municipal government were associated with municipal supportive housing policy. More research should be conducted to complete this data set and further examine the relationship between municipal supportive housing and local governance arrangements.

Table A.3 DUMMY VARIABLES

Variable	FSQCA Conversion	Source	Stata Conversion
Continuum of Care number (local homeless governance system identifier)	U.S. Department of Housing and Urban Development (HUD) identifier		HUD numeric identifier
Continuum of Care name	Name of Continuum of Care by geographic area; HUD Identifier	HUD (2019b)	Text value for identification purposes
State			State identifiers not recoded as numeric value in current dataset; recoded in Stata analyses
FIPS number	Local Geographic Identifier for US Municipalities	U.S. Census Bureau (2018)	Numeric identifier for matching purposes

fsQCA Deduction Procedure

BASELINE ASSUMPTIONS AND HYPOTHESES FOR PATHWAYS IN EACH OUTCOME

This appendix describes the baseline assumptions, informed by existing theory and empirics that advised my approach to running the fsQCA analysis by determining my starting pathways from which I implement the minimization procedure. I describe these assumptions, and then describe procedure used to run fsQCA's stratified, proportional sampling approach that identifies exemplars most predictive and representative of each municipal outcome.

Institutional Resources

For cities *that do not have a municipal level supportive housing policy*, I assumed that limited institutional resources could constrain ability to adopt supportive housing policies. Institutional resources include level of existing infrastructure and financial resources. For example, if a city has low financial resources to support supportive housing sites and services— for example, not expanded Medicaid, low gross domestic product, no state level supportive housing law—the city may not have the fiscal ability to move forward on a supportive housing policy and may default to no action. Municipalities may perceive start-up costs to supportive housing as prohibitively expensive or may perceive inaction on supportive housing and other acute alternatives such as punitive responses as more cost-effective when considering other municipal goals (Nacgourney 2016), adding to perceived cost-effectiveness compared to supportive housing.

Assumptions informing fsQCA procedure:

1. Municipalities *without* a local supportive housing policy are less likely to reside in Medicaid expansion states and states *with* a municipal supportive housing policy.
2. Municipalities *without* a local supportive housing policy are likely to have lower gross domestic product compared to municipalities *with* supportive housing policies.

Political Institutions

In municipalities *without* a local supportive housing policy, I assumed that governmental fragmentation may hinder supportive housing policy adoption. For example, if a city is highly decentralized or very fragmented—with multiple competing municipal jurisdiction—it may be more difficult for actors to engage in local policy processes and to coordinate action. Fragmentation may act as an impediment in this way to adopting supportive housing initiatives. Further, supportive housing actions may be curbed within government itself, if offices and service delivery are decentralized to the degree that it affects intragovernmental coordination. In the same vein, the plurality of municipal governments also affects the ability of constituents to participate in processes (Mickey 2015). Municipal government design interacts with ideology; thus, in more conservative municipal governments, more unilateral systems may close out minority voices arguing for supportive housing policies. Therefore, I assume that municipalities without a supportive housing policy, which are comparatively more conservative, are more likely to have less pluralistic municipal governmental structures. Finally, consistent with the institutional resources assumption, I assumed that municipalities without a supportive housing policy may have fewer delegated state actors providing services and, subsequently, lobbying for supportive housing policies as interest group members, as another challenge for adopting supportive housing policies.

Assumptions informing fsQCA procedure:

1. Municipalities without a supportive housing policy are associated with higher levels of municipal governmental fragmentation compared to cities adopting supportive housing.
2. Municipalities with a supportive housing policy is associated with higher levels of nonprofit healthcare providers compared to cities adopting criminalization only.
3. Municipalities without a supportive housing policy are associated with more unilateral municipal government design in conjunction with more conservative ideology.

Social Construction

Lastly, the way that policy beneficiaries are perceived affects political deliberations over the policies in question (Schneider and Ingram 1993). As proxies for social construction, I assume that more conservative cities with higher percentages of minority groups—Latino and Black—are more likely to not have a municipal level supportive housing policy. The assumption I base this on is the historical literature on vagrancy, deviance, race, and mental illness (Grob 1994). Chronically homeless persons are primarily single men of color. Therefore, municipalities may opt away from welfare policies targeting this population in favor of inaction or other competing policies (such as punitive responses to homelessness). The long history of criminalization of single men of color in the United States, particularly in former confederate states, gives evidence for this assumption. Following from this, I also assume that municipalities without a local supportive housing policy are not likely to be sanctuary cities, as a proxy for local perceptions of immigrations. Low-income immigrant and refugee groups are at higher risks of experiencing homelessness.

Assumptions informing fsQCA procedure:

1. Municipalities without a supportive housing policy are less likely to be sanctuary cities, compared to municipalities with supportive housing policies.
2. Municipalities with higher city-policy conservatism, that are not Sanctuary Cities, and have a higher percentage of minority populations are more likely to be municipalities without a local supportive housing policy.

To begin the analysis, you must input combinations of independent variables to test their collective association with the outcome of interest. With a high number of independent variables, it is impossible to test all possible combinations of conditions. To overcome this limitation, the initial combinations are selected based on the theoretical and empirical literature regarding municipal politics, health policy decision-making, and current municipal homeless policy choices.

Grappling with inherent heterogeneity across cases means that researchers have a tradeoff to make. fsQCA measures pathways based on *coverage* and *consistency*. Coverage is proportion of the sample in the outcome set that adheres to the tested pathway. When evaluating the value of a pathway, coverage matters. Coverage matters because a pathway could exist in 5% of cases or in 50% of cases. The lower the coverage means that the pathway is more of an outlier, reducing the generalizability. The ideal pathway is one that holds predictive value across many or most cases. However, this is where the tradeoff arises. Consistency, as opposed to coverage, measures the degree to which a causal combination leads to an outcome. Within the sample, this means the proportion of cases with the given predictive combination that are also in the outcome set. [1] Due to heterogeneity across individual cases, the greater coverage of a pathway, the lower the consistency, and vice versa—the higher the consistency, the lower the coverage. Having high consistency is a necessity, because we are assuming that the combination leads to the outcome in question. Low consistency violates that assumption and reduces or removes any explanatory power from the pathway. Therefore, depending on the number of variables input into the pathway and the inherent heterogeneity of the sample, researchers must weigh varying degrees of consistency and coverage to reach a predictive and generalizable pathway.

For each outcome, I begin with the combination of independent variables most supported by the literature (as previously stated in my baseline assumptions). Based on the results, I systematically add or subtract variables from the baseline pathway to improve *consistency* and *coverage*. Adding or removing individual variables can notably affect the consistency and coverage of a pathway. Therefore, when initially testing a pathway embedded in the literature, I add or remove single variables at a time to test the overall effect on the pathway. I continue until I reach a threshold for both indicators—unable to further improve coverage and consistency.

Interviewee Demographics by Cases

San Francisco		Shreveport		Atlanta	
Interviewee ID	Interviewee Occupation	Interviewee ID	Interviewee Occupation	Interviewee ID	Interviewee Occupation
1.1	City of San Francisco bureaucrat/ Continuum of Care actor/ homeless services	2.1	Healthcare practitioner	3.1	Municipal service provider/ public safety
1.2	City of San Francisco bureaucrat/ healthcare practitioner	2.2	Continuum of Care actor	3.2	City of Atlanta bureaucrat/ Continuum of Care actor
1.3	Community-based organization (CBO) actor/ homeless services	2.3	Local elected official	3.3	CBO actor homeless services
1.4	City of San Francisco bureaucrat/ government services	2.4	CBO actor/ healthcare services	3.4	City of Atlanta bureaucrat/ government operations

San Francisco		Shreveport		Atlanta	
Interviewee ID	Interviewee Occupation	Interviewee ID	Interviewee Occupation	Interviewee ID	Interviewee Occupation
1.5	City of San Francisco bureaucrat/ healthcare practitioner	2.5	CBO actor/ homeless services	3.5	CBO actor homeless services
1.6	CBO actor/ homeless services	2.6	CBO actor/ healthcare and homeless services	3.6	Academic expert/CBO actor homeless services
1.7	CBO actor/ homeless services	2.7	CBO actor/ low-income services	3.7	Academic expert/CBO actor homeless services
1.8	Academic expert/ healthcare practitioner	2.8	Healthcare practitioner/ academic expert/CBO actor	3.8	Academic expert/ healthcare practitioner
1.9	Municipal service provider/public safety	2.9	CBO actor/ low-income services	3.9	Academic expert/ healthcare practitioner
1.10	Academic expert/ healthcare practitioner/CBO actor	2.10	Service provider/ homeless veterans services	3.10	CBO actor homeless services
1.11	City of San Francisco bureaucrat/ healthcare practitioner	2.11	CBO actor/ low-income services	3.11	City of Atlanta bureaucrat/ government operations
1.12	City of San Francisco bureaucrat/ healthcare practitioner	2.12	Federal actor/inter- government support	3.12	Academic expert/ healthcare practitioner

San Francisco		Shreveport		Atlanta	
Interviewee ID	Interviewee Occupation	Interviewee ID	Interviewee Occupation	Interviewee ID	Interviewee Occupation
1.13	Municipal service provider/ healthcare practitioner	2.13	CBO actor	3.13	Municipal service provider / public safety
1.14	State of California bureaucrat/City of San Francisco bureaucrat/ healthcare practitioner			3.14	Healthcare practitioner
1.15	Municipal service provider/public safety			3.15	Healthcare practitioner
1.16	Municipal service provider/ healthcare practitioner			3.16	Academic expert/City of Atlanta bureaucrat
1.17	Business sector, San Francisco			3.17	CBO actor homeless services
1.18	State of California bureaucrat/City of San Francisco bureaucrat			3.18	City of Atlanta bureaucrat/ homeless services practitioner
				3.19	City of Atlanta bureaucrat/ homeless services practitioner

Qualitative Interview Consent Protocol

Hello, I am a doctoral candidate at the University of Michigan's School of Public Health, in the Department of Health Management and Policy. I am working on my dissertation looking at variation in homeless policy decision-making across the U.S. Thank you for taking time to speak with me.

Before we begin, I want to let you know that this interview is anonymous. All of your identifiable information will be kept anonymous—for example, your name, the names of your department/organization. Only a generic, broad descriptor of your role will be included to identify the sector that you represent—for example, "healthcare practitioner" or "municipal bureaucracy." Only myself and my academic advisors will have access to your identifiable information. This research has been approved by the University Health Sciences Institutional Review Board, and my academic advisors are on the IRB approval along with myself. This interview is not recorded, but I will be taking typed notes. Finally, the interview should take about 30 minutes, but may be shorter or longer depending on your responses. Please let me know if you have any questions or concerns.

Qualitative Interview Questionnaire

1. Could you give me an overview of your role?
2. Please describe the city's current approach to chronic homelessness:
3. Why has the city decided to take this approach?
   A. When was this approach first considered?
   B. Who was involved?
4. From your role, can you provide an overview of how this approach came to be adopted by the city?
   A. What was your role [your department/organization]?
   B. Were there any challenges?
   C. Was there opposition to this policy?
      I. What was the opposition?
      II. Why?
5. Could you speak to the Federal government's position on [city's policy approach]?
   A. Could you discuss the Federal government's role in homelessness/criminalization policy? [e.g. HUD federal incentives to reduce punitive responses to homelessness]
      I. Why?
   B. How has your organization responded to the Federal government's role, how have others in [city] responded?
      I. Why?

II. Was this approach and position considered when deciding the city's approach? Could you describe the federal government's role (if not already discussed)?

C. What about the position of the state? [prompt about Medicaid expansion if not mentioned]

6. Is there any other information that you would like to share?

Codebook for Qualitative Interviews

1. Actor
   a. Municipal bureaucrat
   b. Law enforcement/public safety
   c. Community-based organization/nonprofit staff
   d. Elected official
   e. Healthcare professional
   f. Place of worship
   g. Private/for-profit organization
   h. Tech company
2. City's approach
   a. Defined approach [perceived as having]
   b. Not defined [city perceived to not have a defined approach]
   c. Evidence-based/helpful approached [city perceived to have this]
   d. Nonevidence-based/harmful/less helpful approach [city perceived to have this]
   e. Why approach selected [actor's perception of why city adopted × policy]
   f. Homelessness prioritized [yes/if not don't apply code]
3. Process
   a. Year started
   b. Political will [toward or against supportive housing/addressing homelessness]
      i. Positive [mobilization toward]
   c. Initiating actor

    d. Actors involved overall
       i. Actors not involved [purposefully, or due to institutional barriers/other barriers]
      ii. Participation challenges [inability to participate, limited participation in debates, decision-making]
    e. Process ongoing
       i. Still trying to initiate policy change
      ii. Implementation ongoing
    f. Funding [money to support process/city approach]
       i. City
      ii. State
     iii. Federal
     iv. Community-based organization
      v. Tech/private money
4. Challenges
    a. Coordination challenges
    b. Limited funding
    c. Political pressure on bureaucracy [elected officials pressuring regulators]
    d. Authority/responsibility [authority/responsibility changed, or there is uncertainty about who is responsible]
    e. Stigma
    f. Racial issues
    g. Administrative burden [shift to making it more burdensome for individual to receive government benefits]
    h. Different approaches [different ideas about best approach]
       i. Conflicting approaches/conflicting policies
      ii. Pace [conflicts about pace/timing of policies; conflicting notions of how quick an issue can and should be managed]
     iii. Addressing causes of homelessness vs. homeless behaviors [conflict described between these approaches]
    i. Omitted/underaddressed problems
       i. Food insecurity
      ii. Mental health
     iii. Long-term mental health services
     iv. Housing
5. Opposition
    a. Public/citizens
       i. "Not in my backyard" (NIMBY)
      ii. Gentrification policing
    b. Police/law enforcement

    c. Business/private interests

    d. Other

    e. Elected officials [different ideas/conflicting ideas between elected officials and other groups; pressure, if not direct opposition]

6. Federal involvement [if unsure/not answered, leave blank]

    a. Yes

        i. Effective

        ii. Ineffective

        iii. Future concerns

    b. No

    c. Future concerns [funding/programming/partisanship]

7. Criminalization [law enforcement involvement]

    a. Federal government and local criminalization approach

    b. Local law enforcement response

    c. Law enforcement as service providers

8. State Involvement

    a. State involved

    b. State not involved

    c. State funding

        i. Medicaid expansion funding

    d. Medicaid expansion involved

    e. Medicaid expansion not involved

    f. Challenges with Medicaid expansion implementation

    g. Implementation challenges with state laws

Process Tracing Analytic Approach and for Archival Documents

Starting with the municipal supportive housing policy in each case, I retrospectively searched municipal archives to identify the policy histories behind the adoption of supportive housing policy in each municipality (i.e., events related to the absence of homeless policy in each case) related to responses to homelessness and chronic homelessness in each municipality. This includes relevant state level policies that may have influenced local policy choices. Relevant state level policies were identified based on salience in interviews and local municipal supportive housing policy documents. I organized the policy documents chronologically to establish a sequence of events and temporality in the decision-making processes, triangulating these findings with the interview results. I confirmed data points—timelines and important factors related to decision-making— with multiple sources to confirm or refute the temporality of events and further validate interview findings.

NOTES

ACKNOWLEDGMENTS

1. *Funding disclosure*: Research reported in this publication was supported by the National Institute of Mental Health of the National Institutes of Health under Award Number T32MH019733. The content is solely the responsibility of the authors and does not necessarily represent the official views of the National Institutes of Health.

CHAPTER 1

1. These annual rates of homelessness are not available for persons over age 25. Thus, the estimates included here are a notable undercount by omitting a large proportion of the persons experiencing homelessness who are older, single adults, and the newly increasing population of homeless that includes elderly persons. The coronavirus pandemic of 2020 is associated with dramatically increased rates of homelessness (Tsai and Wilson 2020). The full extent of the influence of coronavirus on rates of homelessness will most likely not be understood for some time but will likely be similar to or probably worse than the Great Recession of 2008.

2. The federal definition of individual, chronic homelessness "refers to an individual with a disability who has been continuously homeless for one year or more or has experienced at least four episodes of homelessness in the last three years where the combined length of time homeless on those occasions is at least 12 months" (U.S. Department of Housing and Urban Development 2019a, 2).

3. Nationally, about one-third of persons experiencing unsheltered homelessness have patterns of chronic homelessness in the United States (U.S. Department of Housing and Urban Development 2019a, 22).

4. Permanent supportive housing provides simultaneous access to both housing and supportive medical and behavioral health services for persons experiencing chronic homelessness. Providing housing allows individuals to feel safe and to access basic needs like sleep, food, and water, promoting an environment where individuals can, subsequently, successfully address chronic medical and behavioral health conditions (Kertesz et al. 2016). Housing First has been the only approach to chronic homelessness that has led to successful, long-term housing stability (M. M. Brown et al. 2016; Leff et al. 2009; Palepu et al. 2013). A recent review by the National Academy of Sciences concluded that Housing First is the best approach to ending chronic homelessness, but it is not clear the degree to which Housing First may improve health outcomes as a result of data/

research design constraints in past research (National Academies of Sciences Engineering and Medicine 2018).

5. These policy changes did not come into effect until the 2016 funding applications. Thus, there is not yet enough data to empirically measure the effect of the 2015 federal regulatory change on municipal policy outcomes.

CHAPTER 2

1. These policy changes did not come into effect until the 2016 funding applications. Thus, there are not yet enough data to empirically measure the effect of the 2015 federal regulatory change on municipal policy outcomes.

CHAPTER 3

1. To receive federal funding, Continuum of Cares are required to use language describing their commitment to promoting evidence-based policies, which may or may not reflect actual change on the ground. Therefore, measuring Continuum of Care policy change may be less valid and may not reflect true policy change or implementation. Further, to design and implement supportive housing policies, municipalities have more political leverage and, potentially, more resources available to them compared to the Continuum of Cares. From zoning to building permitting for shelters or housing units to coordinating police responses to homelessness and county-level health and behavioral health programming to public works for city street clean-up programs (which engage directly with homeless encampments), municipalities hold very high stakes in, and control resources for and implementation of, homelessness policy and programming. As such, measuring municipal policy may more accurately capture street-level policy, as well as leverage for policy change.

2. Therefore, the majority of cities in the United States also align with a county government. So, a Continuum of Care located in one major U.S. city may be aligned with the city and/or county government (e.g., Los Angeles City and Los Angeles County). Since no data currently exist on Continuum of Care governance structures and since Continuum of Cares are an amalgamation of various health delivery systems and actors in a metropolitan area, we cannot delineate between city and county governments as the main governmental partner for Continuum of Cares. Thus, as will be discussed more later in the text, this research assumes that either cities, counties, or both may participate in Continuum of Care governance (if municipal government does participate in Continuum of Care governance) and that supportive housing policy data are collected from cities and counties organized around the local Continuum of Care (e.g., Los Angeles City and Los Angeles County).

3. Sensitivity analyses were also conducted using alternative measure of state policy (presence of state level supportive housing laws) and an alternative measure of the dependent variable local supportive housing policy (number of supportive housing beds) to further test the model and reduce potential measurement error or omitted variable bias. In each case, the sensitivity analyses reduced the predictive power of the model.

4. Set membership to select most representative cases is determined by minimums. Determining membership across two variables takes the minimum of the two scores. Consistency is the sum of the minimum of the membership scores for x and y, over the sum of the minimum membership scores for x. Coverage is

determined by the sum of the minimum of the membership scores for x and y, over the sum of the membership scores for y.

5. Religiosity fell out early in the models, not being consistently predictive or representative. Religiosity was therefore not present as a characteristic in the models although Provo was identified as an exemplar.

6. I encountered unanticipated challenges to recruiting interviewees. Response rates from prospective interviewees was below 25% across the cases. Many prospective interviewees expressed interest, but ultimately declined the request as a result of time constraints. All of the individuals interviewed emphasized substantial time constraints. Ten interviewees had to leave during the interview for another meeting or phone call. The majority of interviewees are both practitioners and policy decision makers. This dual role may have created time constraints that inhibited participation in this study.

CHAPTER 4

1. In the set theoretic analysis, variables from the original dataset "fell out" of the original model that, a priori, would have appeared to be more predictive. These variables include: state level supportive housing policy, tourism, Continuum of Care types, south, former confederacy, etc.; all of the variables not included in the final logit model in Chapter 4. The deduction used in the set theory to sort through which combinations of variables were more or predictive of the outcomes indicates that the variables that "fell out" of the models occur less frequently in the outcome sets, and/or were not predictive.

2. The overall lower rates of minority populations in the most commonly predictive city types may not be an accurate reflection of the relative percentage of people in racial minority groups in these municipalities compared to other municipalities. Municipalities with supportive housing tend to be more diverse on average, but that average diversity is around 20% Black or Latino. Twenty percent—although, on average, a higher percentage of ethnic minority group members—would still be coded as an overall "lower" rate of ethnic minority group members based on set membership. Although the role of race/ethnicity may not be accurately captured in the pathway analysis, the effects of race/ethnicity will be evaluated in the qualitative phase of the research.

3. All control variables were included except for total number of unsheltered chronically homeless (overlap with total chronically homeless) and Continuum of Care type (overlap with metropolitan statistical area size/population) to account for power.

CHAPTER 5

1. U.S. Department of Housing and Urban Development (2017b) defines Continuums of Care as follows: "Continuum of Care and Continuum means the group organized to carry out the responsibilities required under this part and that is composed of representatives of organizations, including nonprofit homeless providers, victim service providers, faith-based organizations, governments, businesses, advocates, public housing agencies, school districts, social service providers, mental health agencies, hospitals, universities, affordable housing developers, law enforcement, organizations that serve homeless and formerly homeless veterans, and homeless and formerly homeless persons to the extent these groups are represented within the geographic area and are available to participate."

2. As mentioned in the Chapter 1, the coronavirus pandemic of 2020 is associated with dramatically increased rates of homelessness (Tsai and Wilson 2020). The full extent of the influence of coronavirus on rates of homelessness will most likely not be understood for some time but will likely be similar to or probably worse than the Great Recession of 2008 (Community Solutions 2020).
3. Whole Person Care (WPC) is an existing Medicaid waiver pursued by the city and county of San Francisco to specifically target chronic homelessness. WPC seeks to align state and local programming to improve coordination and delivery of services to individuals experiencing chronic homelessness. At the time of this research WPC was not implemented, so interviewees could not speak to the effects of WPC on the delivery of services to persons experiencing chronic homelessness and improved policy alignment of state and local efforts to address chronic homelessness.
4. Interviewee 1.8 academic expert/healthcare practitioner.
5. Interviewee 1.3 CBO actor/homeless services.
6. Voluntary in that communities do not have to establish a Continuum of Care yet must establish a Continuum of Care to receive federal funding to address homelessness (U.S. Department of Housing and Urban Development 2017b).
7. Interviewee 1.2 City of San Francisco bureaucrat/healthcare practitioner.
8. Interviewee 1.11 City of San Francisco bureaucrat/healthcare practitioner.
9. Interviewee 1.7 CBO actor/homeless services.
10. Interviewee 1.12 City of San Francisco bureaucrat/healthcare practitioner.
11. Interviewee 1.11 City of San Francisco bureaucrat/healthcare practitioner.
12. Interviewee 1.8 Academic expert/healthcare practitioner.
13. Interviewee 1.11 City of San Francisco bureaucrat/healthcare practitioner.
14. The 311 data updates continuously. This total is the number of calls regarding encampments up until August 5, 2019.
15. Interviewee 1.15 municipal service provider/public safety.
16. San Francisco's Board of Supervisors is San Francisco's city council.
17. There is no available archival documentation of these engagement efforts.
18. Interviewee 1.3 CBO actor/homeless services.
19. Interviewee 1.16 municipal service provider/healthcare practitioner.
20. Interviewee 1.13 municipal service provider/healthcare practitioner.
21. The majority of persons experiencing chronic homelessness have co-occurring mental health and/or substance use disorders.
22. Interviewee 1.2 City of San Francisco bureaucrat/healthcare practitioner.
23. Interviewee 1.10 academic expert/healthcare practitioner/CBO actor.
24. Interviewee 1.11 City of San Francisco bureaucrat/healthcare practitioner.
25. Interviewee 1.15 municipal service provider/public safety.
26. Interviewee 1.3 CBO actor/homeless services.
27. Interviewee 1.6 CBO actor/homeless services.
28. Interviewee 1.11 City of San Francisco bureaucrat/healthcare practitioner.
29. Interviewee 1.8 academic expert/healthcare practitioner.
30. Interviewee 1.12 City of San Francisco bureaucrat/healthcare practitioner.
31. Interviewee 1.12 City of San Francisco bureaucrat/healthcare practitioner.
32. See note 3, this chapter. At the time of this research Whole Person Care (WPC) was not implemented, so interviewees could not speak to the effects of WPC on the delivery of services to persons experiencing chronic homelessness and improved policy alignment of state and local efforts to address chronic homelessness. The year 2017 was a preparation year; 2018 was the start year;

2019 was about making meaningful connections between various services; and 2020 is about evaluation and sustainability. Most interviewees did not discuss WPC, but of those who did most were concerned with ongoing enrollment and coordination issues and the ability of WPC to alleviate those challenges or not. WPC may offer opportunities for policy alignment in the future, which is discussed in the policy implications.

33. Interviewee 1.14 State of California bureaucrat/city of San Francisco bureaucrat/healthcare practitioner.
34. Interviewee 1.8 academic expert/healthcare practitioner.
35. Interviewee 1.1 City of San Francisco bureaucrat/continuum of care actor/homeless services.
36. Interviewee 1.12, City of San Francisco bureaucrat/healthcare practitioner.
37. Funding announcements were listed in January 2019 after California voters passed Proposition 63 to allow for MHSA funds to be used for permanent supportive housing (Department of Housing and Community Development and State of California 2019). The State of California announced funding calls in March but had not yet distributed monies. The funding competition continued through summer 2019 for the first and second rounds.

CHAPTER 6

1. By contrast, alternative counts of homelessness in Atlanta, including the Atlanta Youth Homeless Count and Needs Assessment, estimate 3,374 18- to 25-year-olds in the Atlanta metropolitan area in 2015 and 3,372 in 2018 (Atlanta Youth Count 2015; Giarratano 2019). This count is 20 times higher than the estimates of young adult homelessness counted in the Atlanta Continuum of Care Point-in-Time estimates, including the population counts from DeKalb and Fulton county.
2. Interviewee 3.17 CBO actor.
3. Interviewee 3.4 City of Atlanta bureaucrat, government operations.
4. Interviewee 3.2 City of Atlanta bureaucrat/Continuum of Care actor.
5. Interviewee 3.2 City of Atlanta bureaucrat/Continuum of Care Actor.
6. Interviewee 3.16 academic expert/City of Atlanta bureaucrat.
7. Interviewee 3.18 City of Atlanta bureaucrat/homeless services practitioner.
8. Interviewee 3.7 academic expert/community-based organization (CBO) actor homeless services.
9. Interviewee 3.6 academic expert/CBO actor homeless services.
10. Interviewee 3.7 academic expert/CBO actor homeless services.
11. Interviewee 3.17 CBO actor homeless services.
12. Interviewee 3.19 City of Atlanta bureaucrat/homeless services practitioner.
13. Interviewee 3.6 academic expert/CBO actor homeless services.
14. Interviewee 3.13 municipal service provider—public safety.
15. Interviewee 3.12 academic expert/healthcare practitioner.
16. Interviewee 3.15 healthcare practitioner.
17. Interviewee 3.17 CBO actor homeless services.
18. This search was conducted in 2017, searching Lexis Nexis (now NexisUni) and triangulated against the State of Georgia's legislative database to search for state-level policies addressing homelessness.
19. Interviewee 3.2 City of Atlanta bureaucrat/Continuum of Care actor.
20. Interviewee 3.5 CBO actor homeless services.
21. Interviewee 3.2 City of Atlanta bureaucrat/Continuum of Care actor.

22. Interview 3.16 academic expert/City of Atlanta bureaucrat.
23. Interviewee 3.3 CBO actor homeless services.

CHAPTER 7

1. HOPE for the Homeless Continuum of Care also coordinates homeless services for persons experiencing homelessness outside of Shreveport in the northwest Louisiana area, although Shreveport is their primary population as the area outside of Shreveport is very low population density.
2. Shreveport's archival database and in person records I was able to access is limited to 2002. Interviewees recollection dates back to early 2000s, with more established timelines from 2008 onward.
3. Interviewee 2.2 nonprofit/Continuum of Care stakeholder.
4. Interviewee 2.5 community-based organization (CBO) actor/homeless services.
5. Interviewee 2.7 CBO actor low-income services.
6. Interviewee 2.4 CBO actor.
7. Interviewee 2.8 healthcare practitioner/academic expert/CBO actor.
8. Interviewee 2.7 CBO actor/low-income services.
9. Interviewee 2.4 CBO actor/healthcare services.
10. Interviewee 2.4 CBO actor/healthcare services.
11. Interviewee 2.6 CBO actor homeless services.
12. Interviewee 2.6 CBO actor/healthcare and homeless services.
13. The defined lack of authority by interviewees and archival documents was most often described as "requests" or "asks" for reform or participation by police in trainings and the absence of any "mandate" or "requirement," paired with the described separation of the Continuum of Care from local government.
14. See Chapter 5 of this volume for more details on state approaches to Medicaid and homelessness.
15. Interviewee 2.2 Continuum of Care actor.
16. Interviewee 2.1 healthcare practitioner.
17. Interviewee 2.1 healthcare provider.
18. Interviewee 2.3 local elected official.
19. Interviewee 2.4; healthcare provider.
20. Interviewee 2.1, healthcare practitioner.
21. Interviewee 2.8 CBO actor/healthcare practitioner.

CHAPTER 8

1. *"Continuum of Care and Continuum* means the group organized to carry out the responsibilities required under this part and that is composed of representatives of organizations, including nonprofit homeless providers, victim service providers, faith-based organizations, governments, businesses, advocates, public housing agencies, school districts, social service providers, mental health agencies, hospitals, universities, affordable housing developers, law enforcement, organizations that serve homeless and formerly homeless veterans, and homeless and formerly homeless persons to the extent these groups are represented within the geographic area and are available to participate." (U.S. Department of Housing and Urban Development 2017b)
2. Supportive housing and Housing First pair access to housing with access to supportive medical and social services, addressing both the lack of housing as well as persons physical, behavioral, and social needs. A Housing First approach for supportive housing has been emphasized as since the 1980s, providing access

to housing and supportive services without requiring prerequisites to accessing services such as sobriety. Supportive housing, with a Housing First approach, has now been found over the past few decades to be the most effective method to permanently ending chronic homelessness (National Academies of Sciences Engineering and Medicine 2018; Padgett, Henwood, and Tsemberis 2015).

3. The delegated state is defined as a set of "invisible," or indirect, mechanisms guiding governmental activities and programs for the public through nongovernmental organizations, such as private for profit and nonprofit organizations (Hackett 2017). These invisible mechanisms include governments incentivizing private activity or delivery of certain social services by giving subsidies or benefits to the private organizations via tax subsidies, rebates, and credits (Hackett 2017; Mettler 2011; Morgan and Campbell 2011).

APPENDIX B

1. Set membership is determined by minimums. Determining membership across two variables takes the minimum of the two scores. Consistency is the sum of the minimum of the membership scores for x and y, over the sum of the minimum membership scores for x. Coverage is determined by the sum of the minimum of the membership scores for x and y, over the sum of the membership scores for y.

REFERENCES

Alderwick, Hugh, Carlyn M. Hood-Ronick, and Laura M. Gottlieb. 2019. "Medicaid Investments to Address Social Needs in Oregon and California." *Health Affairs (Project Hope)* 38(5): 774–781.

Anckar, Carsten. 2008. "On the Applicability of the Most Similar Systems Design and the Most Different Systems Design in Comparative Research." *International Journal of Social Research Methodology* 11(5): 389–401.

Anoll, Allison P. 2018. "What Makes a Good Neighbor? Race, Place, and Norms of Political Participation." *American Political Science Review* 112: 494–508.

Applied Survey Research. 2017. *San Francisco Homeless Count & Survey 2017: Comprehensive Report.* www.appliedsurveyresearch.org.

Arno, Peter S. 1986. "The Nonprofit Sector's Response to the AIDS Epidemic: Community-Based Services in San Francisco." *American Journal of Public Health* 76(11): 1325–1330.

Arno, Peter S., and Robert G. Hughes. 1989. "Local Policy Responses to the AIDS Epidemic: New York and San Francisco." In *Acquired Immunodeficiency Syndrome*, eds. P. J. Imperato. Boston, MA: Springer US. 11–19.

Association of Religion Data Archives. 2010. "U.S. Religion Census: Religious Congregations and Membership Study, 2010 (Metro Area File)." U.S. Church Membership Data—County Level. http://www.thearda.com/Archive/Files/Downloads/RCMSMT10_DL2.asp (May 8, 2017).

Atlanta Development Authority. 2008. *2008 ADA Annual Report.* http://lehd.did.census (April 4, 2019).

Atlanta Development Authority. 2009. *2009 Annual Report.* https://www.investatlanta.com/assets/2009_invest_atlanta_annual_report_xD2qEPk.pdf (April 4, 2019).

Atlanta Youth Count. 2015. "AYCNA 2015 Key Findings." *AYCNA 2015 Project Overview.* https://atlantayouthcount.weebly.com/aycna-2015-key-findings.html (July 14, 2020).

Aviram, Uri, and Steven Segal. 1977. "From Hospital to Community Care: The Change in the Mental Health Treatment System in California." *Community Mental Health Journal* 13(2): 158–167.

Bates, Laurie J., and Rexford E. Santerre. 1994. "The Determinants of Restrictive Residential Zoning: Some Empirical Findings." *Journal of Regional Science* 34(2): 253–263.

Bauman, Anna. 2020. "SF Supervisor's CAREN Act Would Make 'False Racially Biased' Calls to Police Illegal." *San Francisco Chronicle*, July 8.

https://www.sfchronicle.com/bayarea/article/SF-supe-proposes-CAREN-Act-to-prohibit-false-15392969.php (July 15, 2020).

Bauman, Tristia et al. 2017. *Housing Not Handcuffs: Ending the Criminalization of Homelessness in U.S. Cities*. Washington, DC: National Law Center on Homelessness and Poverty.

Bayor, Ronald H. 1988. "Roads to Racial Segregation: Atlanta in the Twentieth Century." *Journal of Urban History* 15(1): 3–21.

Bennett, Andrew. 2009. "Process Tracing: A Bayesian Perspective." In *The Oxford Handbook of Political Methodology*, eds. Janet Box-Steffensmeier, Henry E. Brady, and David Collier. New York, NY: Oxford University Press. 1–22.

Bennett, Andrew. 2010. *"Process Tracing and Causal Inference"*. In *Rethinking Social Inquiry : Diverse Tools, Shared Standards*, eds. Henry E. Brady, and David Collier. Lanham, MD: Rowman & Littlefield Publishers. 207–221.

Berkeley Law Policy Advocacy Clinic. 2018. *Homeless Exclusion Districts: How California Business Improvement Districts Use Policy Advocacy and Policing Practices to Exclude Homeless People from Public Space*. Berkeley, CA. https://www.law.berkeley.edu/wp-content/uploads/2018/09/SSRN-id3221446.pdf (March 5, 2020).

Berman, David R. 1997. "State-Local Relations: Devolution, Mandates, and Money." In *The Municipal Year Book*, Washington DC: International City/County Management Association, 40–49.

Berry, Christopher. 2009. *Imperfect Union: Representation and Taxation in Multilevel Governments*. New York, NY: Cambridge University Press.

Bharel, Monica et al. 2013. "Health Care Utilization Patterns of Homeless Individuals in Boston: Preparing for Medicaid Expansion under the Affordable Care Act." *American Journal of Public Health* 103(Suppl. 2): S311–S317.

Biles, Roger. 2011. *The Fate of Cities: Urban America and the Federal Government, 1945-2000*. Lawrence, KS: University Press of Kansas.

Birstow, Miki. 2018. *Navigation Centers: What Do Neighbors Have to Fear?* https://hsh.sfgov.org/wp-content/uploads/2020/01/Navigation-Center-Neighborhood-Impacts-Final-Report-1.pdf (July 6, 2020).

Bishop, Korrin et al. 2017. "The 2017 Annual Homeless Assessment Report (AHAR) to Congress." https://www.hudexchange.info/resources/documents/2017-AHAR-Part-1.pdf (May 7, 2018).

Blair, Thomas R. 2016. "Plague Doctors in the HIV/AIDS Epidemic: Mental Health Professionals and the 'San Francisco Model,' 1981–1990." *Bulletin of the History of Medicine* 90(2): 279–311.

Boston Health Care for the Homeless Program. 2020. "Consumer Advisory Board." *Leadership and Staff*. https://www.bhchp.org/consumer-advisory-board (July 15, 2020).

Bowe, Rebecca. 2015. "S.F. Study Documents Sharp Decline in Mission's Latino Population." *KQED*. https://www.kqed.org/news/10736143/s-f-study-documents-sharp-decline-in-missions-latino-population (May 27, 2019).

Bowers, Melanie. 2015. "Local Policymaking in an Age of Federalism: The Role of Federal Incentives in Municipal Homelessness Policy." PhD diss., Michigan State University.

Brendler, Michael D., and Charlotte A. Jones. 2000. "The Long Run Effect of the Oil Price Collapse on Income Distribution: An Empirical Analysis of Louisiana Metropolitan Areas." *Proceedings of the American Society of Business and Behavioral Sciences*, 7(9): 106–116.

Brescia, Raymond. 2015. "The Criminalization of Mental Illness." *Albany Government Law Review* 8(2): vii–xiv.

Bridges, Amy. 1999. *Morning Glories: Municipal Reform in the Southwest*. Princeton, NJ: Princeton University Press.

Brown, Garrett W, Iain McLean, and Alistair McMillan. 2018. "Tyranny of the Majority." In *A Concise Oxford Dictionary of Politics and International Relations*. eds. Garrett W. Brown, Iain McLean, and Alistair McMillan New York, NY: Oxford University Press.

Brown, Molly M. et al. 2016. "Housing First as an Effective Model for Community Stabilization among Vulnerable Individuals with Chronic and Nonchronic Homelessness Histories." *Journal of Community Psychology* 44(3): 384–390.

Bruff, Harold H. 2010. "Presidential Power Meets Bureaucratic Expertise." *Journal of Constitutional Law* 12(2): 461–490.

Brumble, Melody. 2013. "Help for the Homeless." *The Shreveport Times*. http://proxy.lib.umich.edu/login?url=https://search-proquest-com.proxy.lib.umich.edu/docview/1426037379?accountid=14667.

Bullard, R. D., G. S. Johnson, and A. Torres. 1999. "Atlanta Megasprawl." *Forum for Applied Research and Public Policy* 14(3): 17–23.

Bullard, Robert D., Glenn S. Johnson, and Angel O. Torres, eds. 2000. *Sprawl City : Race, Politics, and Planning in Atlanta*. Washington, DC: Island Press.

Bureau of Economic Analysis. 2017. "GDP and Personal Income." *Regional Data*. https://apps.bea.gov/itable/iTable.cfm?ReqID=70&step=1

Byrne, Hannah. 2018. "The Berkeley Remix, Season Three: First Response—AIDS and Community in San Francisco." *Oral History Review* 45(2): 332–334.

Byrne, Thomas et al. 2014. "The Relationship between Community Investment in Permanent Supportive Housing and Chronic Homelessness." *Social Service Review* 88(2): 234–263.

California Department of Housing and Community Development. 2019. "No Place Like Home Program." *Programs*. http://www.hcd.ca.gov/grants-funding/active-funding/nplh.shtml (May 28, 2019).

California Mental Health Services Oversight and Accountability Commission. 2019. "Proposition 63 History." *History*. https://www.mhsoac.ca.gov/history (May 28, 2019).

Cardinale, Matthew Charles. 2014. "Possible Bribery of Atlanta Official Seen in Special Mater's Ruling in Task Force Lawsuit." *Atlanta Progressive News*, April 12. http://atlantaprogressivenews.com/2014/04/12/possible-bribery-of-atlanta-official-seen-in-special-masters-ruling-in-task-force-lawsuit/

Cassidy, Amanda. 2016. "Medicaid and Permanent Supportive Housing. Medicaid Offers Opportunities to Address Supportive Housing Needs, But Challenges Remain." *Health Affairs*, October 14. https://www.healthaffairs.org/do/10.1377/hpb20161014.734003/full/healthpolicybrief_164.pdf (December 24, 2017).

Centers for Medicare and Medicaid Services. 2019. "State Waivers List." Medaid.gov. https://www.medicaid.gov/medicaid/section-1115-demo/demonstration-and-waiver-list/index.html (August 3, 2019).

Chapin Hall University of Chicago. 2018. *Missed Opportunities: Youth Homelessness in America National Estimates*. http://voicesofyouthcount.org/wp-content/uploads/2017/11/VoYC-National-Estimates-Brief-Chapin-Hall-2017.pdf (December 7, 2018).

Chetty, Raj, Nathaniel Hendren, and Lawrence Katz. 2015. *The Effects of Exposure to Better Neighborhoods on Children: New Evidence from the Moving to Opportunity Experiment*. Cambridge, MA: National Bureau of Economic Research.

Cisneros, Lisa. 2011. "Thirty Years of AIDS: A Timeline of the Epidemic." University of California San Francisco. https://www.ucsf.edu/news/2011/06/9971/thirty-years-aids-timeline-epidemic (May 27, 2019).

City and County of San Francisco. 2010. "San Francisco City and County: Decennial Census Data - 2000-2010." *Bay Area Census*. http://www.bayareacensus.ca.gov/counties/SanFranciscoCounty.htm.

City and County of San Francisco. 2018. "Poverty in San Francisco: Blacks & African American Residents Experience Poverty at 3x the Average Rate." *City Performance Scorecards*. https://sfgov.org/scorecards/safety-net/poverty-san-francisco

City and County of San Francisco. 2019. "311 Cases." *DataSF*. https://data.sfgov.org/City-Infrastructure/311-Cases/vw6y-z8j6 (August 5, 2019).

City and County of San Francisco. 2019. "Homeless Population." *City Performance Scorecards*. https://sfgov.org/scorecards/safety-net/homeless-population (November 25, 2020).

City and County of San Francisco. 2020. "SF Housing Data Hub: Housing Overview." *DataSF*. https://housing.datasf.org/overview/.

City of Atlanta. 2011. "Atlanta, GA : News List : City of Atlanta Awarded $3.3 Million from Bloomberg Philanthropies" [Press release]. https://www.atlantaga.gov/Home/Components/News/News/854/ (April 3, 2019).

City of Atlanta Continuum of Care. 2015. "HUD Exchange: CPD Consolidated Plans, Annual Action Plans, and CAPERs." *Atlanta Consolidated Plan*. https://www.hudexchange.info/programs/consolidated-plan/con-plans-aaps-capers/.

City of Atlanta Innovation Delivery Team. 2014. "Reducing Street Homelessness in Atlanta." *Impact Report*. https://issuu.com/idtatl/docs/atlanta_idt_impact_report_-_reducin (April 2, 2019).

City of San Francisco Department of Public Health. 2000. *HIV/AIDS Epidemiology Annual Report: Department of Public Health HIV Seroepidemiology and AIDS Surveillance Section*. www.dph.sf.ca.us/PHP/AIDSSurvUnit.htm (May 27, 2019).

City of Shreveport, Louisiana. 2014. *Fact Sheet: An Ordinance Declaring the City's Interest in Certain Vacant Property*. Shreveport, LA: City of Shreveport City Council.

City of Shreveport, Louisiana. 2015. *Notice of Public Meeting: July 13, 2015*. Shreveport, LA: City of Shreveport City Council.

City of Shreveport, Louisiana 2016. *HUD Annual Action Plan Funding Year 2015*. Shreveport, LA.

City of Shreveport, Louisiana. 2017. *HUD Annual Action Plan Funding Year 2017*. Shreveport, LA.

City of Shreveport, Louisiana. 2019. "Agendas and Minutes." https://www.shreveportla.gov/AgendaCenter/Search/?term=homeless&CIDs=1,&startDate=&endDate=&dateRange=&dateSelector= (May 9, 2019).

Clifford, Scott, and Spencer Piston. 2017. "Explaining Public Support for Counterproductive Homelessness Policy: The Role of Disgust." *Political Behavior* 39: 503–525.

Cole, Ian. 2006. "Hidden from History? Housing Studies, the Perpetual Present and the Case of Social Housing in Britain." *Housing Studies* 21(2): 283–295.

Collier, David. 2011. "Understanding Process Tracing." *Political Science and Politics* 4: 823–830.

Community Solutions. 2020. "Analysis on Unemployment Projects 40–45% Increase in Homelessness This Year." https://community.solutions/analysis-on-unemployment-projects-40-45-increase-in-homelessness-this-year/ (June 29, 2020).

Conlan, Timothy. 1998. *From New Federalism to Devolution: Twenty-Five Years of Intergovernmental Reform*. Washington, DC: Brookings Institution Press.

Cook, Benjamin L. et al. 2017. "Assessing the Individual, Neighborhood, and Policy Predictors of Disparities in Mental Health Care." *Medical Care Research and Review* 74(4): 404–430.

Cooper, Anastasia. 2013. "The Ongoing Correctional Chaos in Criminalizing Mental Illness: The Realignment's Effects on California Jails." *Hastings Women's Law Journal* 24(2): art. 4.

Council of State Governments. 2013. *Medicaid and Financing Health Care for Individuals Involved with the Criminal Justice System*. Washington, DC. https://csgjusticecenter.org/wp-content/uploads/2013/12/ACA-Medicaid-Expansion-Policy-Brief.pdf (May 9, 2019).

County Behavioral Health Director's Association. 2015. *Mental Health Services Act: History and Orientation*. https://www.cibhs.org/sites/main/files/file-attachments/mon_915_innes_gomberg_history_evolution_of_mhsa.pdf (May 27, 2019).

Cowan, Jill. 2019. "Homeless Populations Are Surging in Los Angeles. Here's Why." *The New York Times*. https://www.nytimes.com/2019/06/05/us/los-angeles-homeless-population.html.

Cronley, Courtney. 2010. "Unraveling the Social Construction of Homelessness." *Journal of Human Behavior in the Social Environment* 20(2): 319–333.

Cubit. 2020. "California Cities by Population." *California Demographics*. https://www.california-demographics.com/cities_by_population (July 6, 2020).

Data USA. 2020a. "Atlanta, GA." https://datausa.io/profile/geo/atlanta-ga (July 7, 2020).

Data USA. 2020b. "San Francisco, CA." https://datausa.io/profile/geo/san-francisco-ca/ (July 6, 2020).

Data USA. 2020c. "Shreveport, LA." https://datausa.io/profile/geo/shreveport-la/ (April 27, 2020).

Davidson, Nestor. 2007. "Cooperative Localism: Federal-Local Collaboration in an Era of State Sovereignty." *Virginia Law Review* 93(4): 959–1034.

Davis, Box 3. 1987. "Hunger/Homeless (6)." OA15701. Washington, DC: Reagan Presidential Library: National Archives and Records Administration.

De Benedictis-Kessner, Justin, and Christopher Warshaw. 2015. "Mayoral Partisanship and the Size of Municipal Government." http://cwarshaw.scripts.mit.edu/papers/CitiesMayors150830.pdf (May 23, 2017).

Deere, Stephen. 2018. "Atlanta Loses $1 Million Federal Grant for Affordable Housing." *Atlanta Journal-Constitution*, December 14. https://www.ajc.com/news/local-govt--politics/atlanta-loses-million-federal-grant-for-affordable-housing/pMSQ9Ug6oIbC8zstdIttxM/

Deere, Stephen. 2019. "Atlanta Council, Mayor at Odds Over Plan to Stem Corruption." *Atlanta Journal-Constitution*, January 28. https://www.ajc.com/news/local-govt--politics/atlanta-council-mayor-odds-over-plan-stem-corruption/RU0uww7u8ojyuv6W9TWhwK/

Deere, Stephen, J. Scott Trubey, and Dan Klepal. 2018. "Bribery Charges Expose Depth of Corruption Facing Atlanta's New Mayor." *Atlanta Journal-Constitution*, April 9. https://www.ajc.com/news/local-govt--politics/bribery-charges-expose-depth-corruption-facing-atlanta-new-mayor/tX8TTszRApqTbor7uTTB2K/

Degeorge, Betsy. 2010. "Migration Patterns of the Homeless Population." *Rescue Magazine*.

Deloitte Consulting. 2003. *Blueprint to End Homelessness in Atlanta in Ten Years*. http://www.hmissummit.net/coc/10 Year Plans/AtlantaGA.pdf (April 3, 2019).

Department of Health, State of Louisiana. 2017. "Permanent Supportive Housing (PSH)." *State of Louisiana*. http://www.dhh.louisiana.gov/index.cfm/page/1732 (September 12, 2017).

Department of Health Care Services, State of California. 2011. *State of California Description of Staff Performing Eligibility Determinations*. https://www.dhcs.ca.gov/formsandpubs/laws/Documents/Attachment 1.2-D.pdf

Department of Health Care Services, State of California. 2019a. "All County Welfare Director's Letters and Medi-Cal Eligibility Division Information Letters." https://www.dhcs.ca.gov/services/medi-cal/eligibility/Pages/ACWDLbyyear.aspx

Department of Health Care Services, State of California. 2019b. *Section 1—Single State Agency*. https://www.dhcs.ca.gov/formsandpubs/laws/Pages/StatePlanDocuments2.aspx.

Department of Health Care Services, State of California. 2020. "Mental Health Services Act." California.gov. https://www.dhcs.ca.gov/services/mh/Pages/MH_Prop63.aspx.

Department of Homelessness and Supportive Housing, San Francisco. 2019a. Navigation Centers Presentation. http://hsh.sfgov.org

Department of Homelessness and Supportive Housing, San Francisco. 2019b. "San Francisco Navigation Centers and SAFE Navigation." *Navigation Centers*. https://hsh.sfgov.org/services/shelter/navigation-centers/ (May 28, 2019).

Department of Homelessness and Supportive Housing and City, San Francisco, and County of San Francisco. 2019. "Local Homeless Coordinating Board." *About Us*. http://hsh.sfgov.org/lhcb/local-homeless-coordinating-board-about-us/ (May 27, 2019).

Department of Housing and Community Development, San Francisco, and State of California. 2019. "California Department of Housing and Community Development Awards $302 Million of No Place Like Home Funds to Help Counties Address Homelessness." Gavin Newsom, Governor. https://www.hcd.ca.gov/about/newsroom/docs/NPLH-Press-Release-Round-1-032019.pdf (July 6, 2020).

Dillon, John F. 1911. *Commentary on the Law of Municipal Corporations*. 5th ed. Boston, MA: Little, Brown.

Diiulio, John J. 2012. "Facing Up to Big Government." *National Affairs*, Spring. https://www.nationalaffairs.com/publications/detail/facing-up-to-big-government

Dillon, Liam. 2018. "$2 Billion to Help House California's Homeless Isn't Being Spent—and No One Knows When It Will Be." *Los Angeles Times*. https://www.latimes.com/politics/la-pol-ca-homeless-housing-bond-stalled-20180301-story.html

Dipietro, Barbara, Samantha Artiga, and Alexandra Gates. 2014. *Early Impacts of the Medicaid Expansion for the Homeless Population.* http://files.kff.org/attachment/early-impacts-of-the-medicaid-expansion-for-the-homeless-population-issue-brief (August 29, 2017).

Dolan, Maura. 2020. "London Breed Pushes San Francisco Reforms: Police No Longer Will Respond to Noncriminal Calls." *Los Angeles Times.* https://www.latimes.com/california/story/2020-06-12/san-francisco-police-reforms-stop-response-noncriminal-calls

Doran, Kelly M., Elizabeth J. Misa, and Nirav R. Shah. 2013. "Housing as Health Care—New York's Boundary-Crossing Experiment." *New England Journal of Medicine* 369(25): 2374–2377.

Dreier, Peter. 2007. "The New Politics of Housing: How to Rebuild the Constituency for a Progressive Federal Housing Policy." *Journal of the American Planning Association* 63(1): 5–27.

Durden, Jada. 2015. "HOPE Expanding Services to Better Help the Homeless." *The Shreveport Times*, April 14. https://www.shreveporttimes.com/story/life/community/2015/04/14/hope-expanding-services-better-help-homeless/25727585/ (August 3, 2019).

Editors of Encyclopaedia Britannica. 2019. "Confederate States of America." *Britannica.* https://www.britannica.com/topic/Confederate-States-of-America (August 1, 2019).

Einstein, Katherine Levine, David M. Glick, and Maxwell Palmer. 2019. *Neighborhood Defenders: Participatory Politics and America's Housing Crisis.* Cambridge, England: Cambridge University Press.

Einstein, Katherine Levine, Maxwell Palmer, and David Glick. 2018. *Racial Disparities in Housing Politics: Evidence from Administrative Data.* https://maxwellpalmer.com/research/racial_disparities_in_housing_politics.pdf (May 27, 2019).

Eisenberg, L. 1988. "The Social Construction of Mental Illness." *Psychological Medicine* 18: 1–9.

Elazar, Daniel. 1991. "Cooperative Federalism." In *Competition Among States and Local Governments: Efficiency and Equity,* eds. Daphne A. Kenyon and John Kincaid. Washington, DC: The Urban Institute, Chapter 4.

Elkin, Stephen L. 2008. "Political Theory and Political Economy." In *The Oxford Handbook of Political Theory,* eds. Dryzek, John S, Honig, Bonnie, Philips, Anne. New York, NY: Oxford University Press. 792–809.

Enos, Gary. 2018. "California Voters Will Have Their Say on Stalled Housing Effort for Homeless." *Mental Health Weekly* 28(27): 1–3.

Eskenazi, Joe. 2019. "San Francisco Needs to Build More Navigation Centers—and Also Needs to Stop Monomaniacally Focusing on Navigation Centers." *Mission Local.* https://missionlocal.org/2019/04/san-francisco-needs-to-build-more-navigation-centers-san-francisco-also-needs-to-stop-monomanically-focusing-on-navigation-centers/.

Evans, Joshua, Damian Collins, and Jalene Anderson. 2016. "Homelessness, Bedspace and the Case for Housing First in Canada." *Social Science and Medicine* 168: 249–256.

Everson, Jeff. 2014. "City Council Agenda–11/11/2014." *City of Shreveport Notice of Public Meeting.* https://www.shreveportla.gov/AgendaCenter/ViewFile/Agenda/_11112014-462?html=true (May 9, 2019).

Fagan, Kevin. 2016. "Homelessness Looks the Same as It Did 20 Years Ago." *San Francisco Chronicle*, June 26. https://projects.sfchronicle.com/sf-homeless/overview/ (May 27, 2019).

Fazel, Seena, John R. Geddes, and Margot Kushel. 2014. "The Health of Homeless People in High-Income Countries: Descriptive Epidemiology, Health Consequences, and Clinical and Policy Recommendations." *The Lancet* 384(9953): 1529–1540.

Federal Emergency Management Agency. 2003. "State Disaster Management Course: Unit 3 Disaster Sequence of Events." *FEMA Training Guide*. https://training.fema.gov/emiweb/downloads/is208sdmunit3.pdf

Fenelon, Andrew et al. 2017. "Housing Assistance Programs and Adult Health in the United States." *American Journal of Public Health* 107(4): 571–578.

Fischer, Frank. 2009. *Democracy and Expertise: Reorienting Policy Inquiry*. Oxford, England: Oxford University Press.

Fracassa, Dominic. 2018. "New Command Center Strives to Tackle Homeless Issues More Quickly in SF." *San Francisco Chronicle*, February 19. https://www.sfchronicle.com/bayarea/article/New-command-center-strives-to-tackle-homeless-12623740.php?psid=78O9g

Fracassa, Dominic. 2019a. "Heated Crowds Pack 2 Meetings about Proposed Navigation Center for the Homeless." *San Francisco Chronicle*, March 13. https://www.sfchronicle.com/bayarea/article/Crowded-meetings-on-new-SF-Navigation-Center-13684149.php

Fracassa, Dominic. 2019b. "SF Supervisors Oppose Wiener's New Housing-Near-Transit Bill, But There's Wiggle Room." *San Francisco Chronicle*, April 4. https://www.sfchronicle.com/bayarea/article/SF-supervisors-oppose-Wiener-s-new-13743143.php

Franklin, Shirley. 2002. *A Vision for Housing in Atlanta: Great Housing in Great Neighborhoods STRATEGIC*. Atlanta, GA. https://www.atlantaga.gov/home/showdocument?id=631 (April 3, 2019).

Frederickson, H. G. 1999. "The Repositioning of American Public Administration." *PS: Political Science and Politics* 32(4): 701–711.

Frey, William H. 1979. "Central City White Flight : Racial and Nonracial Causes Author." *American Sociological Review* 44(3): 425–448.

Fuller, Thomas. 2016. "The Loneliness of Being Black in San Francisco." *The New York Times*, July 21. https://www.nytimes.com/2016/07/21/us/black-exodus-from-san-francisco.html.

Fulton County, Georgia. 2012. *Fulton County Court Improvement Task Force Final Report and Recommendations*. www.georgiacourts.gov (April 6, 2019).

Fulton County, Georgia. 2020. "Cities in Fulton County." *Fulton County Services*. https://www.fultoncountyga.gov/inside-fulton-county/cities-in-fulton-county (July 7, 2020).

Fusaro, Vincent A., Helen G. Levy, and H. Luke Shaefer. 2018. "Racial and Ethnic Disparities in the Lifetime Prevalence of Homelessness in the United States." *Demography* 55: 2119–2128. https://doi.org/10.1007/s13524-018-0717-0

Fusch, Patricia I, and Lawrence R Ness. 2015. "Are We There Yet? Data Saturation in Qualitative Research." *The Qualitative Report How To Article* 20(1): 1408–1416.

Frechtling, Joy. 2002. "An Overview of Quantitative and Qualitative Data Collection Methods." *The 2002 User-Friendly Handbook for Project Evaluation*: 43–62. http://www.nsf.gov/pubs/2002/nsf02057/nsf02057.pdf.

Gailmard, Sean, and John W Patty. 2007. "Slackers and Zealots: Civil Service, Policy Discretion, and Bureaucratic Expertise." *American Journal of Political Science* 51(4): 873–889.

Galster, George. 2012. *Driving Detroit: The Quest for Respect in the Motor City.* Philadelphia: University of Pennsylvania Press.

Gateway Center's Commitment. 2019. "About Us." *Gateway Center: Who We Are.* https://www.gatewayctr.org/about/ (April 3, 2019).

Georgia Public Policy Foundation. 1997. "Atlanta's $250 Million Empowerment Zone Mess: Big Promises Produce Few Results." https://www.georgiapolicy. org/1997/08/atlantas-250-million-empowerment-zone-mess-big-promises-produce-few-results/ (April 3, 2019).

Giarratano, Jennifer French. 2019. "Second Metro Atlanta Homeless Youth Count Suggests Need for Earlier Intervention" [Press release]. Georgia State University. https://news.gsu.edu/2019/12/05/second-metro-atlanta-homeless-youth-count-human-trafficking/ (July 14, 2020).

Glendening, Parris N., and Mavis Mann Reeves. 1984. *Pragmatic Federalism: An Intergovernmental View of American Government.* 2nd ed. Pacific Palisades, CA: Palisades.

Goldman, H. H., and J. P. Morrissey. 1985. "The Alchemy of Mental Health Policy: Homelessness and the Fourth Cycle of Reform." *American Journal of Public Health* 75(7): 727–731.

Goodloe, Shantae. 2015. "HUD Makes 1.9 Billion Dollars in Grants Available for Homeless Programs." HUD Archives: News Releases: Department of Housing and Urban Development Office of Public Affairs. https://archives.hud.gov/news/2015/pr15-116.cfm (December 14, 2017).

Goodman, Christopher B. 2015. "Local Government Fragmentation and the Local Public Sector: A Panel Data Analysis." *Public Finance Review* 43(1): 82–107.

Gorman, Anna, and Harriet Blair Rowan. 2019. "The Homeless Are Dying in Record Numbers on the Streets of L.A." *Kaiser Health News*, April 24. https://khn.org/news/the-homeless-are-dying-in-record-numbers-on-the-streets-of-l-a/

Governing Council of Continuum of Care. 2017. *ClearPath: Atlanta's Five-Year Pan to Make Homelessness Race, Brief, and Non-Recurring.* http://www.gatewayctr.org/wp-content/uploads/2017/10/20170607Partners-for-HOME-Strategic-Plan-Brochure_FINAL.pdf (December 27, 2017).

Grant, Roy et al. 2013. "Twenty-Five Years of Child and Family Homelessness: Where Are We Now?" *American Journal of Public Health* 103(Suppl 2): e1.

Graves, Scott. 2018. *California Budget & Policy Center Proposition 2: Should California Sell Bonds Backed by County Mental Health Funds to Develop Supportive Housing for Homeless Residents With Mental Illness?* California Budget and Policy Center. https://calbudgetcenter.org/blog/proposition-2-should-california-sell-bonds-backed-by-county-mental-health-funds-to-develop-supportive-housing-for-homeless-residents-with-mental-illness/

Gray, Diane, Shirley Chau, Tim Huerta, and Jim Frankish. 2011. "Urban–Rural Migration and Health and Quality of Life in Homeless People." *Journal of Social Distress and the Homeless* 20(1–2): 75–93.

Greenberg, Greg A., and Robert A. Rosenheck. 2008. "Jail Incarceration, Homelessness, and Mental Health: A National Study." *Psychiatric Services* 59(2): 170–177.

Greenwood, Ronni Michelle, Ana Stefancic, and Sam Tsemberis. 2013. "Pathways Housing First for Homeless Persons with Psychiatric Disabilities: Program Innovation, Research, and Advocacy." *Journal of Social Issues* 69(4): 645–663.

Greer, Scott L, Matthias Wismar, and Josep Figueras. 2016. *Strengthening Health System Governance: Better Policies, Stronger Performance*. London, England: Open University Press.

Greer, Scott, Matthias Wismar, Josep Figueras, and Charlotte McKee. 2016. "Governance: A Framework." In *Strengthening Health System Governance: Better Policies, Stronger Performance,* eds. Scott L Greer, Matthias Wismar, and Josep Figueras. Brussels, Belgium: European Observatory on Health Systems and Policies.

Grob, Gerald. 1994. *Mad Among Us*. New York, NY: Simon & Schuster.

Grogan, Colleen M., Sunggeun (Ethan) Park. 2017. "The Racial Divide in State Medicaid Expansions." *Journal of Health Politics Policy and Law* 42(3): 541–572.

Grogan, Colleen M., Phillip M. Singer, and David K. Jones. 2017. "Rhetoric and Reform in Waiver States." *Journal of Health Politics Policy and Law* 42(2): 247–284.

Grossman, Matt, and David A. Hopkins. 2016. *Asymmetric Politics: Ideological Republicans and Group Interest Democrats*. New York, NY: Oxford University Press.

Gustafson, Seth. 2013. "Displacement and the Racial State in Olympic Atlanta 1990–1996." *Southeastern Geographer* 53(2): 198–213.

Hackett, Ursula. 2017. "Theorizing the Submerged State: The Politics of Private Schools in the United States." *Policy Studies Journal* 45(3): 464–489.

Hajnal, Zoltan L., and Jessica Trounstine. 2010. "Who or What Governs? The Effects of Economics, Politics, Institutions, and Needs on Local Spending." *American Politics Research* 38(6): 1130–1163.

Hawthorne, William B. et al. 2012. "Incarceration Among Adults Who Are in the Public Mental Health System: Rates, Risk Factors, and Short-Term Outcomes." *Psychiatric Services* 63(1): 26–32.

Heller, Karen. 2019. "How San Francisco Broke America's Heart." *The Washington Post*. https://www.washingtonpost.com/lifestyle/style/how-san-francisco-broke-americas-heart/2019/05/21/ef9a0ac0-70ea-11e9-9eb4-0828f5389013_story.html?noredirect=on&utm_term=.85b267c3d444.

Henwood, Benjamin F., Leopoldo J. Cabassa, Catherine M. Craig, and Deborah K. Padgett. 2013. "Permanent Supportive Housing: Addressing Homelessness and Health Disparities?" *American Journal of Public Health* 103(Suppl. 2): S188–S192.

Henwood, Benjamin F., Thomas Byrne, and Brynn Scriber. 2015. "Examining Mortality among Formerly Homeless Adults Enrolled in Housing First: An Observational Study." *BMC Public Health* 15(1): 1209.

Hobson, Jeremy. 2019. "How Atlanta Is Streamlining Funding and Targeting the Most Vulnerable to Reduce Homelessness." *WBUR*, February 22. https://www.wbur.org/hereandnow/2019/02/22/atlanta-reduce-homelessness (July 7, 2020).

Hogen-Esch, Tom. 2011. "Fragmentation, Fiscal Federalism, and the Ghost of Dillon's Rule: Municipal Incorporation in Southern California, 1950–2010." *California Journal of Politics & Policy Southern California* 3(1): 1950–2010.

Holland, William Wyatt. 2009. "Who Is My Neighbor? Framing Atlanta's Movement to End Homelessness, 1900–2005." PhD diss., Georgia State University.

Holt, James B., and C. P. Lo. 2008. "The Geography of Mortality in the Atlanta Metropolitan Area." *Computers, Environment and Urban Systems* 32: 149–64.

HOPE Connections. 2003. *Hope for the Homeless Plan to End Homelessness in Northwest Louisiana*. http://www.hmissummit.net/coc/10 Year Plans/ShreveportLA.pdf (May 9, 2019).

HOPE Connections. 2019a. "Statistics/Resources." Northwest Louisiana HOPE Connections. http://www.nwlahope.org/statistics-resources.html (May 7, 2019).

HOPE Connections. 2019b. "Who Are We?" Northwest Louisiana HOPE Connections. http://www.nwlahope.org/who-are-we-.html (May 7, 2019).

Hosmer, David W., and Stanley Lemeshow. 2004. *Applied Logistic Regression*. New York, NY: Wiley-Interscience.

"Housing Beyond Shelter : Novel San Francisco Plan Offers Housing Plus Other Needed Services." 1990. *Los Angeles Times*, July 29. https://www.latimes.com/archives/la-xpm-1990-07-29-op-1201-story.html

Huber, John D., and Charles R. Shipan. 2002. *Deliberate Discretion? The Institutional Foundations of Bureaucratic Autonomy*. Cambridge, England: Cambridge University Press.

Hwang, Jackelyn. 2015. "Pioneers of Gentrification: Transformation in Global Neighborhoods in Urban America in the Late Twentieth Century." *Demography* 53: 189–213.

Insurance Institute for Highway Safety, and Highway Loss Data Institute. 2018. "Fatality Facts." *General Statistics*. http://www.iihs.org/iihs/topics/t/general-statistics/fatalityfacts/state-by-state-overview (August 20, 2018).

Jackson, Kenneth T. 2009. "A Nation of Cities: The Federal Government and the Shape of the American Metropolis." *Annals of the American Academy of Political & Social Science* 626: 11–20.

Jacobs, Keith, and Tony Manzi. 2013. "New Localism, Old Retrenchment: The 'Big Society,' Housing Policy and the Politics of Welfare Reform." *Housing, Theory and Society* 30(1): 29–45.

Jacobs, Sonji, and Anna Torres. 2013. "Mayor Kasim Reed Announces Milestone in 100,000 Homes Campaign 2013 100-Day Challenge" [Press release]. City of Atlanta, GA. https://www.atlantaga.gov/Home/Components/News/News/2154/ (April 3, 2019).

Jarpe, Meghan, Jennifer E. Mosely, and Bikki Tran Smith. 2019. "Understanding the Collaborative Planning Process in Homeless Services: Networking, Advocacy, and Local Government Support May Reduce Service Gaps." *Journal of Public Health Management and Practice* 25(3): 262–269.

Jarvie, Jenny. 2006. "Scandal Stirs Issues of Race in Atlanta." *LA Times*, January 23. https://www.latimes.com/archives/la-xpm-2006-jan-23-na-atlanta23-story.html.

Johnson, William G. 1991. "Housing Policy Under the Reagan Presidency: The Demise of an Iron-Triangle." *Policy Studies Review* 10(4): 69–87.

Jones, Marian Mosher. 2015. "Creating a Science of Homelessness During the Reagan Era." *Milbank Quarterly* 93(1): 139–178.

Kahn, Michael. 2019. "Mapping Downtown Atlanta's Present and Planned Developments." *Curbed: Atlanta*. https://atlanta.curbed.com/maps/downtown-atlanta-developments-map-2018 (April 2, 2019).

Kemp, Donna. 2007. *Mental Health in America: A Reference Handbook*. Santa Barbara, CA: ABC-CLIO.

Kennedy, Ralph C. 1967. "The Short-Doyle Program: Its Past and Its Prospects." *California Medicine* 107(6): 490–495.

Kertesz, Stefan G. et al. 2016. "Permanent Supportive Housing for Homeless People—Reframing the Debate." *New England Journal of Medicine* 375(22): 2115–17. http://www.nejm.org/doi/10.1056/NEJMp1608326 (March 6, 2017).

Kim, Dong Soo. 2000. "Another Look at the NIMBY Phenomenon." *Health & Social Work* 25(2): 146–148.

Kingdon, John. 1990. *Agendas, Alternatives and Public Policies*. New York, NY: HarperCollins.

Kirst, Maritt et al. 2014. "The Promise of Recovery: Narratives of Hope among Homeless Individuals with Mental Illness Participating in a Housing First Randomised Controlled Trial in Toronto, Canada: Table 1." *BMJ Open* 4(3). https://doi.org/10.1136/bmjopen-2013-004379

Koh, Katherine A. et al. 2020. "Health Care Spending and Use Among People Experiencing Unstable Housing in the Era of Accountable Care Organizations." *Health Affairs* 39(2): 214–223.

Kruse, Kevin. 2005. *White Flight: Atlanta and the Making of Modern Conservatism*. Princeton, NJ: Princeton University Press.

Kwak, Nancy H. 2018. "Anti-Gentrification Campaigns and the Fight for Local Control in California Cities." *New Global Studies* 12(1): 9–20.

Lamb, Charles M., and Jim Twombly. 1993. "Taking the Local: The Reagan Administration, New Federalism, and Fair Housing Implementation." *Policy Studies Journal* 21(3): 589–598.

Larimer, Mary E. et al. 2009: "Health Care and Public Service Use and Costs Before and After Provision of Housing for Chronically Homeless Persons with Severe Alcohol Problems." *JAMA* 301(13): 1349–1357.

Lassiter, Matthew D. 2006. *The Silent Majority: Suburban Politics in the Sunbelt South*. Princeton, NJ: Princeton University Press.

Lazar, David. 2017. "SFPD Homeless Outreach." In *Punishing the Poorest: How San Francisco's Criminalization of Homelessness Perpetuates Poverty*. Coalition on Homelessness, Human Rights Center, UC Berkeley School of Law. https://www.sanfranciscopolice.org/sites/default/files/Documents/PoliceCommission/Police Commission120617- Homeless 120617.pdf (May 28, 2019).

Lee, David, and Michael McGuire. 2017. "Intergovernmental Alignment, Program Effectiveness, and U.S. Homelessness Policy." *Publius: The Journal of Federalism* 47(4): 622–47.

Leff, H. Stephen et al. 2009. "Does One Size Fit All? What We Can and Can't Learn From a Meta-Analysis of Housing Models for Persons with Mental Illness." *Psychiatric Services* 60(4): 473–482.

Lerman, Amy E., and Vesla M. Weaver. 2018. "The Carceral State and American Political Development." In *Oxford Handbook of American Political Development*, eds. Richard Valelly, Suzanne Mettler, and Robert Lieberman. New York: Oxford University Press. https://doi.org/10.1093/oxfordhb/9780199697915.013.006

Letelier S., Leonardo. 2005. "Explaining Fiscal Decentralization." *Public Finance Review* 33(2): 155–183.

Lieberherr, Eva, Hans Maarse, and Patrick Jeurissen. 2016. "The Governance of Public-Private Partnerships: Lessons from the United Kingdom and Germany." In *Strengthening Health System Governance: Better Policies, Stronger Performance,* eds. Scott L. Greer, Matthias Wismar, and Josep Figueras. Berkshire, England: European Observatory on Health Systems and Policies. 143–159.

Lillvis, Denise F., and Scott L. Greer. 2016. "Strategies for Policy Success: Achieving 'Good' Governance." In *Strengthening Health System Governance: Better Policies, Stronger Performance*, eds. Scott L. Greer, Matthias Wismar, and Josep Figueras. Berkshire, England: European Observatory on Health Systems and Policies. 57–85.

Louisiana Department of Health. 2017a. "Department of Health and Department of Corrections Team up to Provide Health Care Coverage for Newly Released Offenders." *Healthy Louisiana*. http://ldh.la.gov/index.cfm/newsroom/detail/4170 (August 3, 2019).

Louisiana Department of Health. 2017b. *Justice-Involved Pre-Release Enrollment Program Manual: Healthy Louisiana*. http://ldh.la.gov/assets/medicaid/DOC/JIPEPmanual.pdf (August 3, 2019).

Louisiana Housing Corporation. 2016. *Annual Report*. https://cdn2.hubspot.net/hubfs/4280063/Document Libraries/Public Comments and Notices/Annual Reports/LouisianaHousingCorporation_FY2016_Annual_Report_reduced.pdf (August 3, 2019).

Lublin, David. 2004. *The Republican South: Democratization and Partisan Change*. Princeton, NJ: Princeton University Press.

Lucas, Karen. 2012. "Transport and Social Exclusion: Where Are We Now?" *Transport Policy* 20: 105–113.

Luce, John M. 2013. "A Strange New Disease in San Francisco: A Brief History of the City and Its Response to the HIV/AIDS Epidemic." *Annals of the American Thoracic Society* 10(2): 143–147.

Luker, Kristin. 1996. *Dubious Conceptions: The Politics of Teenage Pregnancy*. Cambridge, MA: Harvard University Press.

Macias, Moki. 2017. *Atlanta/Fulton County Pre-Arrest Diversion Initiative Program Evaluation Request for Proposals*. http://rjactioncenter.org/sites/default/files/files/Eval-RFP-Update3-23.pdf (April 3, 2019).

Mahoney, James, and Kathleen Thelen. 2015. *Advances in Comparative-Historical Analysis*. Cambridge, England: Cambridge University Press.

Maqbool, Nabihah, Janet Viveiros, and Mindy Ault. 2015. *The Impacts of Affordable Housing on Health: A Research Summary*. Washington, DC: Center for Housing Policy.

Masland, Mary C. 1996. "The Political Development of 'Program Realignment': California's 1991 Mental Health Care Reform." *Journal of Behavioral Health Services and Research* 23(2): 170–179.

Matheny, Erin et al. 2013. *A Single Night Counts: Homelessness in Louisiana*. https://static1.squarespace.com/static/53332a2de4b025b2a3c554ca/t/53ecdccde4b04a8ebc02f220/1408031949831/2013+LA+State+Homeless+Census+Report.pdf (August 3, 2019).

Maxmen, Amy. 2019. "The Devastating Biological Consequences of Homelessness." *Nature* 569(7757): 467–468.

Mayor's Innovation Delivery Team, Atlanta, GA. 2014. *Unsheltered No More Initiative*. https://www.csh.org/wp-content/uploads/2014/04/Session3D_Atlanta.pdf (April 3, 2019).

Mazzara, Alicia. 2018. "Trump Plan to Raise Minimum Rents Would Put Nearly a Million Children at Risk of Homelessness." Washington, DC: Center on Budget and Policy Priorities. https://www.cbpp.org/blog/.

trump-plan-to-raise-minimum-rents-would-put-nearly-a-million-children-at-risk-of-homelessness-0 (August 17, 2018).

McGarry, Daniel Tafner. 2008. "The Politics of Homelessness in San Francisco 1988–2002." PhD diss., Stanford University.

McNamara, Robert Hartmann, Charles Crawford, and Ronald Burns. 2013. "Policing the Homeless: Policy, Practice, and Perceptions." *Policing: An International Journal of Police Strategies & Management* 36(2): 357–374.

McNeill, Donald. 2016. "Governing a City of Unicorns: Technology Capital and the Urban Politics of San Francisco." *Urban Geography* 37(4): 494–513.

McNiel, Dale E., Renée L. Binder, and Jo C. Robinson. 2005. "Incarceration Associated With Homelessness, Mental Disorder, and Co-Occurring Substance Abuse." *Psychiatric Services* 56(7): 840–846.

Medicaid and CHIP Payment and Access Commission. 2018. *Medicaid and the Criminal Justice System.* https://www.macpac.gov/wp-content/uploads/2018/07/Medicaid-and-the-Criminal-Justice-System.pdf (August 3, 2019).

Medicaid Reentry Act, H.R. 1329, 116th Congr., 1st Sess. (2019). https://www.congress.gov/116/bills/hr1329/BILLS-116hr1329ih.pdf (May 9, 2019).

Mehrotra, Kartikay, and Eric Larson. 2017. "Trump's Sanctuary Cities Order Blocked by Federal Judge." *Bloomberg Politics*, April 25. https://www.bloomberg.com/news/articles/2017-04-25/trump-s-sanctuary-cities-order-blocked-by-federal-judge (May 9, 2017).

Metraux, Stephen, Dan Treglia, and Thomas P. O'Toole. 2016. "Migration by Veterans Who Received Homeless Services From the Department of Veterans Affairs." *Military Medicine* 181(10): 1212–1217.

Metro Atlanta Chamber. 2020. "Profile of Metro Atlanta: Metro Atlanta Demographics Overview." https://www.metroatlantachamber.com/resources/reports-and-information/executive-profile (July 14, 2020).

Mettler, Suzanne. 2011. *The Submerged State: How Invisible Government Policies Undermine American Democracy.* Chicago, IL: University of Chicago Press.

Mettler, Suzanne. 2016. "The Policyscape and the Challenges of Contemporary Politics to Policy Maintenance." *Perspectives on Politics* 14(2): 369–390.

Michener, Jamila. 2016. "Race, Poverty, and the Redistribution of Voting Rights." *Poverty and Public Policy* 8(2): 106–128.

Michener, Jamila D. 2017a. "How Health Policies Affect Health Equity People, Places, Power: Medicaid Concentration and Local Political Participation." *Journal of Health Politics Policy and Law* 42(5): 865–900.

Mickey, Robert. 2015. *Paths Out of Dixie: The Democratization of Authoritarian Enclaves in America's Deep South, 1944–1972.* Princeton, NJ: Princeton University Press.

Mickey, Robert W. 2008. "The Beginning of the End for Authoritarian Rule in America: *Smith v. Allwright* and the Abolition of the White Primary in the Deep South, 1944–1948." *Studies in American Political Development* 22: 143–182.

Miller, David Young. 2002. *The Regional Governing of Metropolitan America.* Boulder, CO: Westview Press.

Mirabal, Nancy Raquel. 2009. "Geographies of Displacement: Latina/Os, Oral History, and the Politics of Gentrification in San Francisco's Mission District." *Source: The Public Historian* 31(2): 7–31.

Monkkonen, Paavo, and Will Livesley-O'Neill. 2017. "Overcoming Opposition to New Housing." UCLA Lewis Center for Regional Policy Studies. https://www.lewis.ucla.edu/opposition-to-new-housing/

Mor, Vincent, John A. Fleishman, John D. Piette, and Susan M. Allen. 1993. "Developing AIDS Community Service Consortia." *Health Affairs Grantwatch*, 12(1): 186–199.

Morewitz, Mark. 2018. "A Brief History of the San Francisco Health Commission." San Francisco Health Commission. https://www.sfdph.org/dph/hc/History2.pdf (July 7, 2020).

Morgan, Kimberly J., and Andrea Louise Campbell. 2011. *The Delegated Welfare State: Medicare, Markets, and the Governance of Social Policy*. Oxford University Press.

Morrissey, J. P., and H. H. Goldman. 1984. "Cycles of Reform in the Care of the Chronically Mentally Ill." *Hospital Community Psychiatry* 35: 785–793.

Moynihan, Donald, Pamela Herd, and Elizabeth Ribgy. 2016. "Policymaking by Other Means: Do States Use Administrative Barriers to Limit Access to Medicaid?" *Administration & Society* 48(4): 497–524.

Mulvey, Philip, and Michael White. 2013. "The Potential for Violence in Arrests of Persons with Mental Illness." *Policing: An International Journal of Police Strategies & Management* 37(2): 404–419.

Municode. 2020. "Library." Municode Library. https://library.municode.com/ (July 2, 2020).

Nacgourney, Adam. 2016. "Aloha and Welcome to Paradise. Unless You're Homeless." *New York Times*, June 4. https://www.nytimes.com/2016/06/04/us/hawaii-homeless-criminal-law-sitting-ban.html

National Academies of Sciences Engineering and Medicine. 2018. *Permanent Supportive Housing : Evaluating the Evidence for Improving Health Outcomes among People Experiencing Chronic Homelessness*. Washington, DC: National Academies Press.

National Center for Charitable Statistics. 2018. "US Nonprofit Sector Publications, Reports and Statistics." https://nccs.urban.org/data-statistics/us-nonprofit-sector-publications-reports-and-statistics (August 21, 2018).

National Centers for Environmental Information and National Oceanographic and Atmospheric Administration. 2017. "Statewide Temperature Mapping: Climate at a Glance." https://www.ncdc.noaa.gov/cag/statewide/mapping/110/tavg/201701/1/value (August 17, 2018).

National Coalition for the Homeless. 2006. "McKinney–Vento Act." NCH Fact Sheet #18. http://www.nationalhomeless.org/publications/facts/McKinney.pdf (December 1, 2015).

National Conference of State Legislatures. 2018. "Affordable Care Act Medicaid Expansion." http://www.ncsl.org/research/health/affordable-care-act-expansion.aspx (August 21, 2018).

"National Homeless Awareness Week." 1986. Reagan Presidential Library: National Archives and Records Administration, Box 69. Washington, DC.

National Institute on Drug Abuse. 2018. "Opioid Overdose Crisis." https://www.drugabuse.gov/drugs-abuse/opioids/opioid-overdose-crisis#five (August 8, 2018).

National Law Center on Homelessness and Poverty. 2015. *Homelessness in America: Overview of Data and Causes*. https://nlchp.org/wp-content/uploads/2018/10/Homeless_Stats_Fact_Sheet.pdf (January 11, 2017).

Padgett, Deborah K., Benjamin F. Henwood, and Sam Tsemberis. 2015. *Housing First: Ending Homelessness, Transforming Systems, and Changing Lives*. New York, NY: Oxford University Press.

Page, Edward C. 2006. "The Origins of Policy." In *The Oxford Handbook of Public Policy*, eds. Michael Moran, Martin Rein, Robert E. Goodin. Oxford, England: Oxford University Press. 207–226.

Palepu, Anita et al. 2013. "Housing First Improves Residential Stability in Homeless Adults with Concurrent Substance Dependence and Mental Disorders." *American Journal of Public Health* 103(Suppl 2): e30–e36.

Paradise, Julia, and Donna Cohen Ross. 2017. *Linking Medicaid and Supportive Housing: Opportunities and On-the-Ground Examples*. Kaiser Family Foundation Issue Brief. http://files.kff.org/attachment/Issue-Brief-Linking-Medicaid-and-Supportive-Housing-Opportunities-and-On-the-Ground-Examples (March 7, 2018).

Parker, R. David, and Shana Dykema. 2013. "The Reality of Homeless Mobility and Implications for Improving Care." *Journal of Community Health* 38(4): 685–689.

Parker, Travis, and Patricia A. Griffin. 2017. *Sequential Intercept Model Mapping Report for Fulton County, GA*. https://www.fultonstepsup.org/sites/default/files/fulton_county_ga_sim_report-_final_with_appendices.pdf (April 6, 2019).

Partners for Home. 2017. *Creating a Clear Path for Atlanta's Homeless*. Georgia State Senate. http://www.senate.ga.gov/committees/Documents/Cathryn_Marchman-Partners_for_HOME.pdf (April 3, 2019).

Pearce, John L. et al. 2016. "Characterizing the Spatial Distribution of Multiple Pollutants and Populations at Risk in Atlanta, Georgia." *Spatial and Spatio-temporal Epidemiology* 18: 13–23. http://dx.doi.org/10.1016/j.sste.2016.02.002

Pendered, David. 2013. "Atlanta's New Answer to Reducing Homelessness: Create a Non-Profit Organization under Mayor's Control." *Saporta Report*. https://saportareport.com/atlantas-new-answer-to-homelessness-create-a-non-profit-under-mayors-control/ (April 3, 2019).

Penner, Susan. 1995. "An Evolving Managed Care System: Public Mental Health Services in San Francisco." *Administration and Policy in Mental Health* 22(3): 273–287.

Perez, Alina, Steven Leifman, and Ana Estrada. 2003. "Reversing the Criminalization of Mental Illness." *Crime and Delinquency* 49(1): 62–78.

Peterson, Paul E. 1981. *City Limits*. Chicago, IL: University of Chicago Press.

Piat, Myra. 2000. "The Nimby Phenonmenon: Community Residents' Concerns about Housing for Deinstitutionalized People." *Health & Social Work* 25(2): 127–138.

Pierson, Paul. 1993. "When Effect Becomes Cause: Policy Feedback and Political Change." *World Politics* 45(4): 595–628.

Pierson, Paul. 1995. "Fragmented Welfare States: Federal Institutions and the Development of Social Policy." *Governance* 8(4): 449–478.

Plümper, Thomas, Vera E. Troeger, and Eric Neumayer. 2019. "Case Selection and Causal Inferences in Qualitative Comparative Research." *PLOS ONE* 14(7): e0219727.

Policy Link, Program for Environmental and Regional Equity, and University of Southern California. 2015. An Equity Profile of the San Francisco Bay Area Region https://www.policylink.org/sites/default/files/documents/bay-area-profile/BayAreaProfile_21April2015_Final.pdf (May 27, 2019).

Poremski, Daniel, Rob Whitley, and Eric Latimer. 2014. "Barriers to Obtaining Employment for People with Severe Mental Illness Experiencing Homelessness." *Journal of Mental Health* 23(4): 181–185.

Pre-Arrest Diversion Design Team. 2017. *Atlanta/Fulton County Pre-Arrest Diversion Initiative*. http://citycouncil.atlantaga.gov/Home/ShowDocument?id=210 (April 3, 2019).

Prioleau, Brian. 2013. "JFK's Legacy of Community-Based Care." Washington, DC: Substance Abuse and Mental Health Services Administration. https://www.samhsa.gov/homelessness-programs-resources/hpr-resources/jfks-legacy-community-based-care (May 27, 2019).

Ragin, Charles. 2015. "Fuzzy Set/Qualitative Comparative Analysis." *fsQCA Introduction*. http://www.u.arizona.edu/~cragin/fsQCA/ (May 10, 2017).

Ragin, Charles C. 2014. *The Comparative Method: Moving Beyond Qualitative and Quantitative Strategies*. Berkeley, CA: University of California Press.

Ragin, Charles C., Kriss A. Drass, and Sean Davey. 2006. "Fuzzy-Set/Qualitative Comparative Analysis 2.0." Tucson, AZ: Department of Sociology, University of Arizona.

Rahaim, John et al. 2018. San Francisco Housing Needs and Trends Report. *San Francisco Planning*. https://sfplanning.org/project/san-francisco-housing-needs-and-trends-report

Rankin, Nicolas R. et al. 2015. "Marta Service Cuts in Hotlanta: Using the Regime Theory and the Environmental Justice Framework to Analyze Transportation Racism in Hotlanta." *Race, Gender & Class* 22(3–4): 55–82.

Rauh, Virginia A., Philip J. Landrigan, and Luz Claudio. 2008. "Housing and Health: Intersection of Poverty and Environmental Exposures." *Annals of the New York Academy of Sciences* 1136: 276–288.

Reed, Kasim. 2014. "Atlanta Reduces Homeless Population (and Saves Money in the Process)." *CNN Business*, December 11. https://money.cnn.com/2014/12/11/news/economy/atlanta-kasim-reed-innovation/index.html (April 3, 2019).

Rinker, Brian. 2019. "Finding Shelter and Support Along the Road to Better Health." *Health Affairs* 38(8): 1252–1256.

Robinson, Tony. 2019. "No Right to Rest: Police Enforcement Patterns and Quality of Life Consequences of the Criminalization of Homelessness." *Urban Affairs Review* 55(1): 41–73. https://doi.org/10.1177/1078087417690833

Rochefort, David A. 1984. "Origins of the 'Third Psychiatric Revolution': The Community Mental Health Centers Act of 1963." *Journal of Health Politics, Policy and Law* 9(1): 1–30.

Rosenbaum, Sara, Sara Schmucker, Sara Rothenberg, and Rachel Gunsalus. 2016. *Streamlining Medicaid Enrollment: The Role of the Health Insurance Marketplaces and the Impact of State Policies*. Washington, DC. https://www.commonwealthfund.org/publications/issue-briefs/2016/mar/streamlining-medicaid-enrollment-role-health-insurance (February 20, 2020).

Ross, Bernhard H., and Myron A. Levine. 2001a. "Formal Structure and Leadership Style." In *Urban Politics: Power in Metropolitan America*, eds. Bernhard H. Ross and Myron A. Levine. Itasca, IL: Peacock. 131–173.

Ross, Bernhard H., and Myron A. Levine. 2001b. "National and State Policy Toward Cities." In *Urban Politics: Power in Metropolitan America*, eds. Bernhard H. Ross and Myron A. Levine. Itasca, IL: Peacock. 441–443.

Roy, Laurence et al. 2016. "Predictors of Criminal Justice System Trajectories of Homeless Adults Living with Mental Illness." *International Journal of Law and Psychiatry*, 49(Pt A):75–83.

Rubin, Herbert J, and Irene S Rubin. 2011. *Qualitative Interviewing: The Art of Hearing Data*. Thousand Oaks, CA: SAGE Publications.

Saks, Elyn R. 2013. "The Status of Status Offenses: Helping Reverse the Criminalization of Mental Illness." *Southern California Review of Law and Social Justice* 23(3): 367–386.

San Francisco Budget and Legislative Analyst's Office. 2016. *Performance Audit of Homeless Services in San Francisco*. Department of Homelessness and Supportive House, June 13. http://hsh.sfgov.org/wp-content/uploads/2016/06/Homeless-Services-in-SF-BLA-Report-June-13-2016.pdf (May 27, 2019).

San Francisco Department of Planning. 2018. *San Francisco Housing Needs and Trends Report Planning Department*. http://www.sfplanning.org (May 27, 2019).

San Francisco Department of Public Health. 2006. *Housing Needs and Current Housing Resources Allocation*. https://www.sfdph.org/dph/files/mtgsGrps/HIVAIDSHousingGrp/files/HousingNeedsyAllocation10032006SL.pdf (May 27, 2019).

San Francisco Department of Public Health. 2017. *Whole Person Care California Medi-Cal 2020 Waiver*. https://www.sfdph.org/dph/hc/HCAgen/HCAgen2017/April 18/2017AprilWPCOverviewISCv041017handoutofpresentation.pdf (October 1, 2018).

San Francisco Department of Public Health. 2019. *San Francisco Mental Health Services Act (MHSA) 2018–19 Annual Report*. https://www.sfdph.org/dph/files/CBHSdocs/MHSAdocs/FY2018-2019MHSA-Annual-Update.pdf (May 27, 2019).

San Francisco Department of Public Health, HIV Seroepidemiology Surveillance Section. 1998. *Annual AIDS Surveillance Report 1998*. https://www.sfdph.org/dph/files/reports/RptsHIVAIDS/HIVAIDAnnlRpt1998.pdf (July 6, 2020).

Saporta, Maria. 2011. "Atlanta Mayor Kasim Reed Establishes 'Innovation Delivery Team' with Bloomberg Funds." *Saporta Report*. https://saportareport.com/atlanta-mayor-kasim-reed-establishes-innovation-delivery-team-with-bloomberg-funds/ (April 3, 2019).

Scheffler, R., A. Zhang, and L. Snowden. 2001. "The Impact of Realignment on Utilization and Cost of Community-Based Mental Health Services in California." *Administration and Policy in Mental Health* 29(2): 129–143.

Scheffler, Richard M., and Neal Adams. 2005. "Millionaires and Mental Health: Proposition 63 in California." *Health Affairs* 24(Suppl 1): W5-212–W5-224.

Schneider, Anne, and Helen Ingram. 1993. "Social Construction of Target Populations: Implications for Politics and Policy." *American Political Science Review* 87(2): 334–347.

Segal, Andrea G., Rosemary Frasso, and Dominic A. Sisti. 2018. "County Jail or Psychiatric Hospital? Ethical Challenges in Correctional Mental Health Care." *Qualitative Health Research* 28(6): 963–976. https://doi.org/10.1177/1049732318762370

Sellers, Jeffrey M. 2002. *Governing from Below: Urban Regions and the Global Economy*. Cambridge, England: Cambridge University Press.

Shadish, W R. 1984. "Policy Research: Lessons from the Implementation of Deinstitutionalization." *American Psychologist* 39(7): 725–738.

Sheperd, Joyce. 2013. *13-R-3111*. Atlanta City Council. http://atlantacityga.iqm2.com/Citizens/Detail_LegiFile.aspx?Frame=&MeetingID=1239&MediaPosition=3666.000&ID=2087&CssClass= (April 3, 2019).

Sherman, John. 2000. "Empowerment Zone: Boondoggle or Aid to Poor?" *Atlanta Business Chronicle*, November 6. https://www.bizjournals.com/atlanta/stories/2000/11/06/editorial5.html (April 3, 2019).

Shipan, Charles R. 2006. "Bottom–Up Federalism: The Diffusion of Antismoking Policies from U.S. Cities to States." *American Journal of Political Science* 50(4): 825–843.

Shreveport Downtown Development Authority. 2019. "Hope for the Homeless: Downtown Development Authority." https://downtownshreveport. com/projects-and-initiatives/hope-for-the-homeless/ (May 9, 2019).

Sisco, Tauna. 2017. "Gender and Policy Implementation: Analyzing and Predicting the Progress of Congressional Bills Targeting Homeless Women." *Journal of Women, Politics, and Policy*, 38(3): 38–408.

Sisti, Dominic A., Andrea G. Segal, and Ezekiel J. Emanuel. 2015. "Improving Long-Term Psychiatric Care: Bring Back the Asylum." *Journal of the American Medical Association* 313(3): 243–244.

Skocpol, Theda, and Paul Pierson. 2007. *The Transformation of American Politics: Activist Government and the Rise of Conservatism*. Princeton, NJ: Princeton University Press.

Smith, Anna V. 2020. "There's Already an Alternative to Calling the Police." *High Country News*. https://www.hcn.org/issues/52.7/public-health-theres-already-an-alternative-to-calling-the-police (July 15, 2020).

Smith, Doug. 2016. "Anti-Homeless Laws Proliferate." *Los Angeles Times*, August 31. http://documents.latimes.com/study-california-anti-homeless-laws/.

Smothers, Ronald. 1996. "As Olympics Approach, Homeless Are Not Feeling at Home in Atlanta." *New York Times*, July 1. https://www.nytimes.com/1996/07/01/ us/as-olympics-approach-homeless-are-not-feeling-at-home-in-atlanta.html (March 30, 2019).

Snowden, Lonnie, Richard Scheffler, and Amy Zhang. 2002. "The Impact of Realignment on the Client Population in California's Public Mental Health System." *Administration and Policy in Mental Health* 29(3): 229–241.

Snyder, Elizabeth. 2016a. "Medicaid and Prisoner Reentry: Suspension Is the New Black." *Journal of Law and Public Policy* 26: 84–104.

Sommers, B. D. et al. 2016. "Insurance Churning Rates for Low-Income Adults Under Health Reform: Lower Than Expected But Still Harmful for Many." *Health Affairs* 35(10): 1816–1824.

Soss, Joe, Richard C. Fording, and Sanford. Schram. 2011. *Disciplining the Poor : Neoliberal Paternalism and the Persistent Power of Race*. Chicago, IL: University of Chicago Press.

Stafford, Amanda, and Lisa Wood. 2017. "Tackling Health Disparities for People Who Are Homeless? Start with Social Determinants." *International Journal of Environmental Research and Public Health* 14(12): 1535.

Stanhope, Victoria, and Kerry Dunn. 2011. "The Curious Case of Housing First: The Limits of Evidence Based Policy." *International Journal of Law and Psychiatry* 34(4): 275–282.

State Health Access Data Assistance Center, Division of Health Policy and Management, and University of Minnesota School of Public Health. 2018. *Assessment and Synthesis of Selected Medicaid Eligibility, Enrollment, and Renewal Processes and Systems in Six States. Medicaid and CHIP Payment and Access Commission (MACPAC)*. https://www.macpac.gov/publication/assessment-and-synthesis-of-selected-medicaid-eligibility-enrollment-and-renewal-processes-and-systems-in-six-states/ (May 9, 2019).

Stergiopoulos, Vicky et al. 2015. "Effectiveness of Housing First with Intensive Case Management in an Ethnically Diverse Sample of Homeless Adults with Mental Illness: A Randomized Controlled Trial." *PLOS ONE* 10(7): e0130281.

Stokes, Stephannie. 2019. "Super Bowl: Atlanta's Pledge to Clear Homeless Camps Fuels Anxiety." National Public Radio, January 31. https://www.npr.org/2019/01/31/690514220/atlantas-pledge-to-clear-homeless-camps-fuels-anxiety-ahead-of-super-bowl (March 30, 2019).

Strach, Patricia. 2015. *Hiding Politics in Plain Sight: Cause Marketing, Corporate Influence, and Breast Cancer Policymaking*. New York, NY: Oxford University Press.

Stringfellow, Erin J. et al. 2016. "Substance Use Among Persons with Homeless Experience in Primary Care." *Substance Abuse* 37(4): 534–541.

Sugrue, Thomas J. 2014. *The Origins of the Urban Crisis: Race and Inequality in Postwar Detroit*. Princeton, NJ: Princeton University Press.

Suzuki, Tami J. 2012. *Finding Aid to the Art Agnos Papers, 1977–2002 (Bulk 1984–1991)*. http://pdf.oac.cdlib.org/pdf/csf/sfpl/agnos.pdf (July 6, 2020).

Takahashi, Lois M. 1997. "The Socio-Spatial Stigmatization of Homelessness and HIV/AIDS: Towards an Explanation of the NIMBY Syndrome." *Social Science and Medicine* 45(6): 903–914.

Tars, Eric. 2015. *The Cost of Criminalizing Homelessness Just Went Up by $1.9 Billion: HUD Funding Requirement Building on Department of Justice Enforcement*. National Law Center on Homelessness and Poverty, September 18. https://www.nlchp.org/press_releases/2015.09.18_HUD_NOFA_criminalization (August 5, 2016).

Tatum, Jason. 2013. "Partner Spotlight: Regional Commission on Homelessness." Gateway Center. https://www.gatewayctr.org/2013/07/partner-spotlight-regional-commission-on-homelessness/ (April 3, 2019).

Editorial Board. 2018. "California's Mental Health Services Act a Good Idea Poorly Executed." *Orange County Register*, March 9. https://www.ocregister.com/2018/03/09/californias-mental-health-services-act-a-good-idea-poorly-executed/ (May 28, 2019).

Torres, Anne, and Jenna Garland. 2017. "Atlanta, GA : News List : Mayor Kasim Reed Announces $50 Million Homeless Opportunity Bond to Move Forward" [Press release]. City of Atlanta, GA. https://www.atlantaga.gov/Home/Components/News/News/6042/1338?backlist=%2F (April 3, 2019).

Torres, Anne, and Jenna Garland. 2018. "Mayor Keisha Lance Bottoms Signs Cash Bond Ordinance into Law" [Press release]. City of Atlanta, GA, February 6. https://www.atlantaga.gov/Home/Components/News/News/11448/1338?backlist=%2525252F (April 3, 2019).

Trounstine, Jessica. 2008. *Political Monopolies in American Cities. The Rise and Fall of Bosses and Reformers*. Chicago, IL: University of Chicago Press.

Trounstine, Jessica. 2019. *Segregation by Design: Local Politics and Inequality in American Cities*. Cambridge, England: Cambridge University Press.

Trounstine, Jessica. 2020. "The Geography of Inequality: How Land Use Regulation Produces Segregation." *American Political Science Review* 114(2): 443–455.

Tsai, Jack, and Michal Wilson. 2020. "COVID-19: A Potential Public Health Problem for Homeless Populations." *The Lancet: Public Health* 5(4): e186–e187.

Tsai, Jack, and Robert A. Rosenheck. 2012. "Incarceration Among Chronically Homeless Adults: Clinical Correlates and Outcomes." *Journal of Forensic Psychology Practice* 12(4): 307–324.

Tsai, Jack, Robert A. Rosenheck, Dennis P. Culhane, and Samantha Artiga. 2013. "Medicaid Expansion: Chronically Homeless Adults Will Need Targeted

Enrollment and Access to a Broad Range of Services." *Health Affairs* 32(9): 1552–1559.

UC San Francisco Library Archives and Calisphere. n.d. "AIDS Substance Abuse Program." *UCSF AIDS Health Project Records*. https://calisphere.org/item/dfd47b0f-1e78-4cf6-9306-63f0e629388b/

U.S. Census Bureau. 2012a. 2012 Census of Governments—Organization. "Data." https://www.census.gov/data/tables/2012/econ/gus/2012-governments.html (August 21, 2018).

U.S. Census Bureau. 2012b. Local Governments in Individual County-Type Areas. *American FactFinder*. https://factfinder.census.gov/faces/tableservices/jsf/pages/productview.xhtml?src=bkmk (August 21, 2018).

U.S. Census Bureau. 2017. "Population Estimates." *U.S. Census Quick Facts*. https://www.census.gov/quickfacts/fact/table/US/PST045219 (November 22, 2020).

U.S. Census Bureau. 2018. 2017 FIPS codes. https://www.census.gov/geographies/reference-files/2017/demo/popest/2017-fips.html

U.S. Department of Commerce Economics and Statistics Administration. 2010. "Census Regions and Divisions of the United States." https://www2.census.gov/geo/pdfs/maps-data/maps/reference/us_regdiv.pdf (October 15, 2017).

U.S. Department of Health and Human Services Assistant Secretary for Planning and Evaluation, and Office of Disability Aging and Long-Term Care Policy. 2014. *Medicaid and Permanent Supportive Housing for Chronically Homeless Individuals: Emerging Practices from the Field*. http://aspe.hhs.gov/daltcp/reports/2014/EmergPrac.pdf

U.S. Department of Health and Human Services Assistant Secretary for Planning and Evaluation, and Office of Disability Aging and Long-Term Care Policy. 2018. *Aging, Reentry, and Health Coverage: Barriers to Medicare and Medicaid for Older Reentrants*. https://aspe.hhs.gov/office-disability-aging (May 10, 2019).

U.S. Department of Housing and Urban Development. 2009. "The McKinney–Vento Homeless Assistance Act as Amended by S. 896 the Homeless Emergency Assistance and Rapid Transition to Housing (HEARTH) Act of 2009." https://www.hudexchange.info/resources/documents/HomelessAssistanceActAmendedbyHEARTH.pdf (November 16, 2017).

U.S. Department of Housing and Urban Development. 2012. *Introductory Guide to the Continuum of Care (CoC) Program*. https://www.hudexchange.info/resources/documents/CoCProgramIntroductoryGuide.pdf (April 6, 2019).

U.S. Department of Housing and Urban Development. 2014. *Citizen Participation and Consultation Toolkit*. https://www.hudexchange.info/onecpd/assets/File/eCon-Planning-Suite-Citizen-Participation-Toolkit.pdf (May 28, 2019).

U.S. Department of Housing and Urban Development. 2015a. *Coordinated Entry Policy Brief*. https://www.hudexchange.info/resources/documents/Coordinated-Entry-Policy-Brief.pdf.

U.S. Department of Housing and Urban Development. 2015b. *Homeless Populations and Subpopulations State Name: GA-502 Fulton County CoC*. HUD Exchange. https://www.hudexchange.info/programs/coc/coc-homeless-populations-and-subpopulations-reports/

U.S. Department of Housing and Urban Development. 2015c. *Homeless Populations and Subpopulations State Name : GA-508 DeKalb County CoC*. HUD Exchange. https://files.hudexchange.info/reports/published/CoC_PopSub_CoC_GA-508-2019_GA_2019.pdf

U.S. Department of Housing and Urban Development. 2015d. "HUD 2015
Continuum of Care Homeless Assistance Programs Homeless Populations and
Subpopulations GA-500 Atlanta CoC." https://files.hudexchange.info/reports/
published/CoC_PopSub_CoC_GA-500-2015_GA_2015.pdf (July 7, 2020).

U.S. Department of Housing and Urban Development. 2015e. "HUD 2015
Continuum of Care Homeless Assistance Programs Homeless Populations
and Subpopulations: CA-501 San Francisco CoC." *HUD Exchange*. https://files.
hudexchange.info/reports/published/CoC_PopSub_CoC_CA-501-2015_CA_
2015.pdf (July 7, 2020).

U.S. Department of Housing and Urban Development. 2015f. "HUD 2015
Continuum of Care Homeless Assistance Programs Homeless Populations and
Subpopulations: Shreveport." *HUD Exchange*. https://files.hudexchange.info/
reports/published/CoC_PopSub_CoC_LA-502-2015_LA_2015.pdf (July 7,
2020)./

U.S. Department of Housing and Urban Development. 2016. "Housing First in
Permanent Supportive Housing." *HUD Exchange*. https://www.hudexchange.
info/resources/documents/Housing-First-Permanent-Supportive-Housing-
Brief.pdf (March 6, 2017).

U.S. Department of Housing and Urban Development. 2017a. "HUD Publishes
Coordinated Entry Requirements and Checklist of Essential Elements–
HUD Exchange." *HUD Exchange*. https://www.hudexchange.info/news/
hud-publishes-coordinated-entry-requirements-and-checklist-of-essential-
elements/ (October 25, 2018).

U.S. Department of Housing and Urban Development. 2017b. "Part 578—Continuum
of Care Program." *Code of Federal Regulations*. https://www.govinfo.gov/
content/pkg/CFR-2017-title24-vol3/xml/CFR-2017-title24-vol3-part578.xml.

U.S. Department of Housing and Urban Development. 2017c. "PIT and HIC Data
Since 2007." *HUD Exchange*. https://www.hudexchange.info/resource/3031/
pit-and-hic-data-since-2007/ (December 30, 2017).

U.S. Department of Housing and Urban Development. 2018a. "Homeless Populations
and Subpopulations: GA-502 Fulton County CoC." *HUD Exchange*. https://files.
hudexchange.info/reports/published/CoC_PopSub_CoC_GA-502-2018_GA_
2018.pdf (July 7, 2020).

U.S. Department of Housing and Urban Development. 2018b. "Homeless Populations
and Subpopulations: GA-508 DeKalb County CoC." *HUD Exchange*. https://
files.hudexchange.info/reports/published/CoC_PopSub_CoC_GA-508-2018_
GA_2018.pdf (July 7, 2020).

U.S. Department of Housing and Urban Development. 2018c. "HUD 2018 Continuum
of Care Program Funding Awards: CoC Name: Shreveport, Bossier/Northwest
Louisiana CoC." *HUD Exchange*. https://files.hudexchange.info/reports/
published/CoC_AwardComp_CoC_LA-502-2018_LA_2018.pdf (February
13, 2020).

U.S. Department of Housing and Urban Development. 2018d. "HUD 2018
Continuum of Care Homeless Assistance Programs Homeless Populations
and Subpopulations GA-500 Atlanta CoC." *HUD Exchange*. https://files.
hudexchange.info/reports/published/CoC_PopSub_CoC_GA-500-2018_GA_
2018.pdf (July 7, 2020).

U.S. Department of Housing and Urban Development. 2018e. "HUD 2018
Continuum of Care Homeless Assistance Programs Homeless Populations
and Subpopulations: CA-501 San Francisco CoC." *HUD Exchange*. https://files.

hudexchange.info/reports/published/CoC_PopSub_CoC_CA-501-2018_CA_
2018.pdf (July 6, 2020).

U.S. Department of Housing and Urban Development. 2018f. "HUD 2018
Continuum of Care Homeless Assistance Programs Homeless Populations
and Subpopulations LA-502 Shreveport, Bossier." *HUD Exchange*. https://
www.hudexchange.info/programs/coc/coc-homeless-populations-and-
subpopulations-reports/.

U.S. Department of Housing and Urban Development. 2018g. "The 2018 Annual
Homeless Assessment Report to Congress Part 1: Point-In-Time Estimates of
Homelessness." *HUD Exchange*. https://www.hudexchange.info/resources/
documents/2012-AHAR-Volume-2-Section-3.pdf.

U.S. Department of Housing and Urban Development. 2019a. "The 2019 Annual
Homeless Assessment Report (AHAR) to Congress." https://www.huduser.gov/
portal/sites/default/files/pdf/2019-AHAR-Part-1.pdf (February 20, 2020).

U.S. Department of Housing and Urban Development. 2019b. "FY 2019 Continuums
of Care Names and Numbers." *HUD Exchange*. https://www.hudexchange.info/
resource/5790/fy-2019-continuums-of-care-names-and-numbers/ (August
5, 2019).

U.S. Department of Housing and Urban Development. 2019c. "CPD Consolidated
Plans, Annual Action Plans, and CAPERs." *HUD Exchange*.

U.S. Department of Housing and Urban Development. 2020. "HMIS Regulations
and Notices." *HUD Exchange*. https://www.hudexchange.info/programs/hmis/
hmis-regulations-and-notices/ (February 4, 2019).

U.S. Department of Housing and Urban Development Office of Policy
Development and Research. 2018. "Coordinating Community Planning."
HUD Exchange https://www.hudexchange.info/resources/documents/
CoordinatingCommPlanning_Presentation.pdf.

U.S. Department of Justice Office of Justice Programs. 2011. "Bureau of Justice
Statistics: National Prisoner Statistics, 1978–2011." *Inter-University Consortium
for Political and Social Research*. https://doi.org/10.3886/ICPSR34540.v1

U.S. Immigration and Customs Enforcement. 2017a. *Enforcement and Removal
Operations: Weekly Detainer Outcome Report for Recorded Declined Detainers Feb
11-Feb 17 2017*. https://www.ice.gov/doclib/ddor/ddor2017_02-11to02-17.pdf
(May 17, 2017).

U.S. Immigrations and Customs Enforcement. 2017b. *Enforcement and Removal
Operations: Weekly Declined Detainer Outcome Report for Recorded Declined
Detainer Outcome Report*. https://www.ice.gov/doclib/ddor/ddor2017_02-
11to02-17.pdf (March 19, 2019).

U.S. Interagency Council on Homelessness. 2015. *Federal Strategic Plan to Prevent
and End Homelessness: Opening Doors*. https://www.hudexchange.info/
resource/1237/usich-opening-doors-federal-strategic-plan-end-homelessness/
(September 24, 2018).

U.S. Interagency Council on Homelessness. 2018. *Homelessness in America: Focus
on Families with Children*. https://www.usich.gov/resources/uploads/asset_
library/Homeslessness_in_America_Families_with_Children.pdf (September
24, 2018).

United Way Atlanta. 2017. *Mission United*. https://www.unitedwayatlanta.org/
program/mission-united/pdf/ (April 3, 2019).

University of California Berkeley School of Law Human Rights Center. 2017.
Punishing the Poor: How San Francisco's Criminalization of Homelessness

Perpetuates Poverty. https://www.sanfranciscopolice.org/sites/default/files/Documents/PoliceCommission/Police Commission120617- Homeless 120617.pdf

University of California Los Angeles. n.d. *Funding Public Mental Health in California.* http://histpubmh.semel.ucla.edu/sites/default/files/story-flipbooks/funding_publicmental_health/files/dmh_funding.pdf (May 27, 2019).

Urban Institute, and Thomas G. Kingsley. 2017. *Trends in Housing Problems and Federal Housing Assistance.* Washington, DC. https://www.urban.org/sites/default/files/publication/94146/trends-in-housing-problems-and-federal-housing-assistance.pdf (May 28, 2019).

Valero, Jesus N., and Hee Soun Jang. 2016. "The Role of Nonprofit Organizations in Homeless Policy Networks: A Research Note." *Cityscape: A Journal of Policy Development and Research* 18(2): 151–162.

Vanneman, Megan E., and Lonnie R Snowden. 2015. "Linking the Legislative Process to the Consequences of Realigning California's Public Mental Health System." *Administration and Policy in Mental Health and Mental Health Services Research* 42: 593–605.

Vogelsang-Coombs, Vera. 2007. "Mayoral Leadership and Facilitative Governance." *The American Review of Public Administration* 37(2): 19–26.

Volk, Jennifer S. et al. 2016. "Tenants with Additional Needs: When Housing First Does Not Solve Homelessness." *Journal of Mental Health* 25(2): 169–175.

Wagner, Robin. 2017. "Louisiana Permanent Supportive Housing." In *NASHP Annual Conference 2017.* https://nashp.org/wp-content/uploads/2017/06/R-Wagner-19.pdf (May 10, 2019).

Walker, David B. 1995. *The Rebirth of Federalism: Slouching Towards Washington.* New York, NY: Chatham House.

Walker, Willie, Dee Dee Kramer, Katherine Ets-Hokin, and Tim Wilson. 1997. *Finding Aid to the San Francisco Department of Public Health AIDS Office Records.* http https://oac.cdlib.org/findaid/ark:/13030/c8833r08/entire_text/ (May 27, 2019).

Ware, Dazara, and Deborah Dennis. 2013. *Best Practices for Increasing Access to SSI/SSDI upon Exiting Criminal Justice Settings.* Substance Abuse and Mental Health Service Administration. http://www.mentalhealthamerica.net (August 19, 2019).

Warfield, Matt, Barbara DiPietro, and Samantha Artiga. 2016. *How Has the ACA Medicaid Expansion Affected Providers Serving the Homeless Population: Analysis of Coverage, Revenues, and Costs.* Henry J. Kaiser Family Foundation. http://www.kff.org/medicaid/issue-brief/how-has-the-aca-medicaid-expansion-affected-providers-serving-the-homeless-population-analysis-of-coverage-revenues-and-costs/ (August 29, 2017).

Warshaw, Chris, and Chris Tausanovitch. 2015. "Replication Data for: Representation in Municipal Government." https://dataverse.harvard.edu/dataset.xhtml?persistentId=doi:10.7910/DVN/AXVEXM (September 24, 2017).

Watson, Sara, and Alison Klurfeld. 2011. *California's Mental Health System.* http://www.ibhpartners.org/wp-content/uploads/2015/12/Mental_Health_Report.pdf (July 6, 2020).

Waxmann, Laura. 2019. "Wiener's Housing Density Legislation Faces Hometown Opposition." *San Francisco Examiner*, March 30. https://www.sfexaminer.com/news/wieners-housing-density-legislation-faces-hometown-opposition/

Weaver, Vesla M. 2007. "Frontlash: Race and the Development of Punitive Crime Policy." *Studies in American Political Development* 21(2): 230–265.

Weicher, J. C. 1984. *Maintaining the Safety Net: Income Redistribution Programs in the Reagan Administration.* Washington, DC: American Enterprise Institute for Public Policy Research.

Weir, Margaret, Ana S Orloff, and Theda Skocpol. 1988. *The Politics of Social Policy in the United States.* Princeton University Press. https://press.princeton.edu/books/paperback/9780691028415/the-politics-of-social-policy-in-the-united-states (September 19, 2020).

Weir, Margaret, and Jessica Schirmer. 2018. "America's Two Worlds of Welfare: Subnational Institutions and Social Assistance in Metropolitan America." Perspectives on Politics 16(2): 380–399.

White, Randol. 2018. "Proposition 2: At Issue Is Housing for 20,000 Mentally Ill Homeless People in California." Sacramento State Capital Public Radio, October 18. http://www.capradio.org/articles/2018/10/18/proposition-2-at-issue-is-housing-for-20000-mentally-ill-homeless-people-in-california/ (May 28, 2019).

Whittle, Henry J. et al. 2015. "Food Insecurity, Chronic Illness, and Gentrification in the San Francisco Bay Area: An Example of Structural Violence in United States Public Policy." *Social Science & Medicine* 143: 154–161. https://doi.org/10.1016/j.socscimed.2015.08.027

WHORM File, and Box 43. 1987. "FITH." Reagan Presidential Library: National Archives and Records Administration.

WHSOF Box 3, and Dan Crippen. 1987. "Memorandum to Domestic Policy Council." Reagan Presidential Library: National Archives and Records Administration.

WHSOF Davis. n.d. "House Committee Summary of Findings." Reagan Presidential Library: National Archives and Records Administration: Box 5.

Willison, Charley. 2017. "Shelter from the Storm: Roles, Responsibilities, and Challenges in United States Housing Policy Governance." *Health Policy* 121: 1113–1123.

Willison, Charley E. 2020. "Local Supportive Housing Policy by Continuum of Care." Harvard Dataverse. https://doi.org/10.7910/DVN/JUWDWY

Witkin, David, and Kaylin Huang. 2018. "Proposition 2: Use Millionaire's Tax Revenue for Homelessness Prevention Housing Bonds Measure." *California Initiative Review* 2018: art. 3.

Wright, James D., Beth A. Rubin, and Joel A. Devine. 1998. *Beside the Golden Door: Policy, Politics, and the Homeless.* New York, NY: Aldine de Gruyter.

Young, Michael G., and Kathleen Manion. 2017. "Harm Reduction through Housing First: An Assessment of the Emergency Warming Centre in Inuvik, Canada." *Harm Reduction Journal* 14(1): art. 8.

Zannoni, Paolo. 1978. "The Concept of Elite." *European Journal of Political Research* 6: 1–30.

Zhang, Amy, Richard Scheffler, and Lonnie Snowden. 2000. "The Effects of Program Realignment on Severely Mentally Ill Persons in California's Community-Based Mental Health System." *Psychiatric Services* 51(9): 1103–1106.

Zlotnick, Cheryl, Suzanne Zerger, and Phyllis B. Wolfe. 2013. "Health Care for the Homeless: What We Have Learned in the Past 30 Years and What's Next." *American Journal of Public Health* 103(Suppl 2): S199–S205.

INDEX

For the benefit of digital users, indexed terms that span two pages (e.g., 52–53) may, on occasion, appear on only one of those pages.

Tables are indicated by *t* following the page number.